PRAISE FOR *LONGEVITY DECODED*

"Dr. Schimpff explores the exciting topic of healthy aging. He combines the science of aging with evidence to suggest how each of us influences our personal journey in life. We make choices every day which impact our health. This book will help you understand how those daily choices will influence your life not only today, but as you get older. Begin today to plan for tomorrow."
—*James (Jim) M. Anders, Jr., CPA, MBA, CGMA, President and Chairman of the Board, National Senior Campuses, Inc., Administrator and Chief Operating Officer, Kennedy Krieger Institute, Inc.*

"A highly enjoyable and uplifting read written by a physician with uncommon intellect and wisdom. Certainly, we can all benefit from following Dr. Schimpff's prescription for a healthier and more meaningful life."
—*R. Alan Butler, Chief Executive Office, Erickson Living*

"Brilliant work by Dr. Stephen Schimpff yet again! Dr. Schimpff has done a systematic analysis of aging and longevity. His uncanny ability to use data and science together makes his suggestions compelling and convincing, while being insightful. Despite being a complete and thorough account for advanced readers, his book is simple enough to understand for a beginner. If there is only *one* book you want to read on this subject, it should be this one."
—*Hiren Doshi, CEO, Paragon Private Health, Co-founder and President, OmniActive Health Technologies*

"The old adage goes 'the only sure things are taxes and aging.' Not so fast! Reading Stephen Schimpff's fascinating new book did not help me pay my taxes, and despite his sage advice, my birthday still came and went. But the concepts he describes (in a meaningful and fun way) made me recognize that the age I feel is truly in my hands!"
—*Stephen K. Klasko, M.D., M.B.A., President and CEO, Thomas Jefferson University and Jefferson Health*

D1593518

"We are witnessing the marketization of a backward behemoth—the U.S. Healthcare industry. Consumers will become a force in a new health economy that will demand clarity, transparency, choice and value. Seniors, already a major social and cultural force in our country, expect more from our healthcare system, and how we transform health for seniors will be central to how we develop the broader roadmap of market reform that is required to improve the health status of all Americans. A big driver is the creation of incentives for healthcare consumers to engage in their healthiness. Aging is not trivial, and it's not a spectator sport, despite what the American medical complex has led us to believe. Dr. Schimpff describes not only what we should expect as we age, but what is expected, and how our taking a more activist role in managing our health is a critical part of a maturing market."
—*Don McDaniel, CEO, Canton & Company, Baltimore, Maryland*

"With remarkable ease and with clarity of message, Dr. Schimpff demystifies the aging process and our current understanding. Most importantly he provides a simple, successful path to realizing your personal goals of health and well-being. As he remarks, '*You can do it.*'"
—*Matt Narrett, MD, Chief Medical Officer, Erickson Living*

"As my age cohort heads toward Medicare, like a veritable tsunami of aging boomers, this text ought to be our navigational guide in the storm. We will want yoga on the lawn, rather than a wheelchair in the garden; we will crave gourmet organic meals, not a nursing home tray!! Dr Schimpff will help us to achieve these dreams with his folksy and reassuring style. This book only confirms for me that the best is yet to come!"
—*David B. Nash MD, MBA. Founding Dean of the Jefferson College of Population Health*

"In this easy to understand, yet frank and direct treatise intended for both patients and physicians, Dr. Stephen Schimpff successfully demystifies human longevity and its relationship to genetics and related environmental factors. He shows how the new primary care paradigm, variously known as direct primary care or concierge care or retainer-based care, allows for close relationships to form between physicians and their patients, which in turn facilitates the creation of customized and personalized health and wellness solutions to extend patient longevity. The 'keys' to a long healthy life revealed by Dr. Schimpff make it a must read for people young and old.

—*Guru Ramanathan Ph.D., Chief Innovation Officer, GNC*

"As the world's older population continues to expand at an unprecedented rate, Dr. Schimpff gives readers simple steps that can lay the crucial groundwork for our future health. He provides an optimistic approach to the inevitability of aging and a refreshing perspective that our 'golden years' can also be our 'golden age,' based on his first-hand experience as a healthcare practitioner."

—*E. Albert Reece, MD, PhD, MBA, Vice President for Medical Affairs, University of Maryland, John Z. and Akiko K. Bowers Distinguished Professor and Dean, University of Maryland School of Medicine*

"We are living longer, but not necessarily better. Societal anti-aging biases are deeply held, reinforcing negative stereotypes about a time in life that should be defined by respect and opportunity. Longevity Decoded challenges this stereotype, offering an alternative perspective to aging that is not only positive but empowering. It is sorely needed in a society that is rapidly aging."

—*Katie Smith Sloan, President and CEO, LeadingAge*

Other books by Dr. Schimpff for a general audience:

The Future of Medicine: Megatrends in Healthcare

Alignment: The Key to the Success of the University of Maryland Medical System

The Future of Healthcare Delivery:
Why it must Change and How it Will Affect You

Fixing the Crisis in Primary Care:
Reclaiming the Patient-Physician Relationship and Returning
Healthcare Decisions to You and Your Doctor

Fortune Seekers in the Promised Land:
A Tale of Exploitation and Development in the Canaan
Valley and Blackwater Region of West Virginia

LONGEVITY DECODED

LONGEVITY DECODED

The 7 KEYS to Healthy Aging

Stephen C Schimpff, MD, MACP

Copyright 2018 Stephen C Schimpff, MD MACP

Published by Squire Publishing, Catonsville, MD

No part of this publication may be reproduced, stored in retrieval system, or transmitted in any form or by any means, electronic, mechanical, photocopying, or recording, scanning, or otherwise, except as permitted under Section 107 or 108 of the 1976 United States Copyright Act, without the prior written permission of the Publisher. Requests to Publisher for permission should be addressed to: schimpff3@gmail.com

ISBN: 978-0-692-06420-7

This book is for educational purposes and is not personal medical or health advice. Please consult with your physician regarding any of the information contained herein. The content of this book is not meant to replace diagnosis or treatment by a competent medical practitioner. While the author has made a concerted effort to provide accurate information, neither the publisher nor author shall have any liability or responsibility for any adverse effects or loss caused, or alleged to be caused, directly or indirectly by any information included in this book.

August, watercolor by Carol Schimpff

Cover design by Lou Moriconi, www.loumoriconi.com

For

My parents,
Donald and Lorraine Schimpff.
They lived life to the fullest and
never let age quell their enthusiasm.

My wife and soulmate,
Carol.
She always inspires me.

Our daughter and son-in-law,
Becky Schimpff and Brian Kushnir.
They make us proud.

Our grandsons,
Ben and Bruno Kushnir.
They give us joy.

TABLE OF CONTENTS

PREFACE

Every year you celebrate a new birthday and each year you are a year older. Your biological clock is ticking. You probably would like to live a long time. You undoubtedly want to be healthy and hope to remain so throughout your lifetime. There are specific actions that you can take to assure that long healthy life. I call them "keys" but there is nothing out of the ordinary about them; indeed, they are very ordinary. These keys tend to be "secret" because so few people know them and fewer still practice them. The price is right; they cost not a penny.

Sure, even with the best of efforts, an unexpected disease can appear, one that medical science is at a loss to prevent or cure. But so many of the diseases that afflict the citizens of Western industrialized countries can be prevented such as heart disease, diabetes, many cancers, strokes, autoimmune diseases, even the most dreaded of all—Alzheimer's disease. If you prevent these, you can have that long and enjoyable life. Remember, your doctor can not do it for you. There is no fountain of youth, at least not yet, and there is no pill to prevent disease and prolong life, again, not yet. So, it is entirely up to you.

You can go into any grocery store, drugstore or health store and see rows of bottles of vitamins, minerals and supplements. And then there are protein mixes, energy drinks and all manner of other prepared and processed foods to consider. Move onto the cosmetic store where you will find many varieties of anti-aging skin creams along with cover-up powders. At the dermatologist you can get Botox. At the plastic surgeon you can get a nip and a tuck or even a full facelift. There are hair transplants, breast implants, and liposuction. There are no anti-aging drugs, but there are prescription medications that will assist you to regain some of your lost abilities from the past.

Or, at no cost, you can follow the time-tested recommendations in this book. The downside is that they will require your full participation. No pills, no surgery, no injections—just constant attention. The keys are all about what you eat and drink, how you move your body and never smoke, how you manage your stress levels and get a good night's sleep. It is also about how you stimulate your brain and keep socially engaged. It sounds easy, but of course it takes your full cooperation and commitment. It will probably be a significant change from what you are doing now, and it may well mean giving up some of your favorite habits. Consider these recommendations when you are still young, before the clock winds down too far. Just like a retirement investment that compounds over the years, attending to these suggestions and recommendations will pay off handsomely down the road of life. But for those of you further down the path, it is never too late to get started; now is the perfect time no matter your age.

My wife's uncle, John Litwin, died last year just short of age 102. He lived the life showcased in this book. Always a good weight for his height – never a "beer belly" – he enjoyed good food but not too much; always active yet slept soundly; had a remarkable ability to never let adversity cause long-term stress; enjoyed time with friends and relatives, and sought out new adventures. He clearly felt comfortable with the life he lived. Still independent and active until Hurricane Sandy put a tree through the roof of his living room, he then moved to an assisted living facility at the urging of his grandsons. When asked his preference for his 98th birthday, he suggested a party at the local bowling alley. Holding a full size, full-weight ball, he walked up to the line, swung his arm back and forth a few times and let the ball go. It moved slowly down the alley; most of us were sure it would roll into the gutter or just stop before it got to the pins. We were all wrong: he had a spare and his score for the afternoon was as good as anyone one third his age and well experienced. We saw him for the last time on Christmas Eve 2015, about eleven months before he died. We had a long conversation with him. He was stone deaf, but technology allowed us to talk and have our words pop up on a screen immediately, so it was nearly a normal conversation. He was crystal clear albeit a bit slow to speak, remembered his time in the Civilian Conservation Corp, the Navy and the torpedoing of his ship, along with more recent activities like fishing with his great grandkids. Asked why he always seemed never stressed, he answered that "I guess I just let it roll off my back." He had a spirit about life and a sense of purpose. I will refer to him a few times as the book proceeds.

This book starts with an overview of the normal aging process and including how it unfolds at a cellular level. There is a look at the new understanding of the biological clocks in our bodies. We then examine those communities around the world that tend to live an exceptionally long time with good health. With this background, we then delve into the specifics of what you can and should do to prevent disease and add quality years to your life. Given that some of you already have a chronic illness or may develop one, we also take a look at how these diseases need to be addressed by you and your healthcare team – quite different from the usual approach to modern medicine. We might term it a paradigm change from 20th century to 21st century healthcare.

Now understanding what you can do, we will nevertheless consider ongoing attempts to find a pill to slow the aging process and how some people are working to actually defy aging with gene therapy. There is a discussion of combating the ever present anti-age bias of society followed by a look at a few philosophical concepts. These round out our understanding of the aging process and our critical and personal role in maintaining our bodies and our brains for the long term because, in the end, it comes down to what you do individually and collectively to foster your health and wellness. Those are the keys. You can then decode them for your own health and longevity.

May you enjoy a long and healthy life, with a deep sense of fulfillment.

Stephen C Schimpff, MD MACP
January, 2018

CHAPTER ONE

INTRODUCTION: THE TRUTH ABOUT AGING

We are all aging every day but mostly we ignore it, do not recognize it, or deny it. Then all of a sudden, we look in the mirror and realize that older age has found us. Even then each person deals with aging differently. In this book we will look at the aging process, some of the known underlying biological mechanisms that drive aging, how we as individuals can slow the aging process, principally using life style modifications, and take a look at some of the research into drugs that might offer a benefit. We will review some of the ongoing attempts to truly defy aging—to find the Fountain of Youth using today's science and technology.

The following poem by an unknown author is a parody of Dr Seuss' classic *The Cat in the Hat*:

I cannot see
I cannot pee
I cannot chew
I cannot screw
Oh, my God, what can I do?
My memory shrinks
My hearing stinks
No sense of smell
I look like hell
My mood is bad—can you tell?
My body's drooping
Have trouble pooping

> The Golden Years have come at last
> The Golden Years can kiss my ass

In this poem, the presumed *The Cat in the Hat* takes a negative perspective on aging. Perhaps the author says much of what many people feel and think.

But there are other perspectives, many much more positive.

When I told a friend about the concept of this book, he sent me the following: "About 25 years ago, I received a video about the Adirondack Park. When the park was established – in the late 1800s I believe – the New York state government drew a blue line around the immense region. Individuals living inside the park were allowed to stay and pass their land onto heirs, but they could not sell their property to others. Over the succeeding generations the land not passed on to heirs became owned by the state. The video was about a gentleman in his sixties who was one of the last of his generation and focused on preserving what had been the Adirondack way of life—realizing it was about to fade into history. In the video, as he talked he slowly unfolded a 6-foot wooden ruler. He went on to indicate that the 72 inches represented the average lifespan in years for many folks. He then indicated his age on the ruler and made the point that while he hoped to live beyond the end of the ruler, he realized his time was short and he had limited time to accomplish his goals.

"My dad had recently passed away – at the age of 72 – and in his tools I found a folding ruler. After seeing the video, I picked up the ruler and unfolding it became aware I was beyond the half way point. Over the years I have often opened and looked at the ruler. I recall at 50 feeling that time was speeding up. For some reason now that I'm in my sixties, the passage of time bothers me less—but I am aware of the limited amount left. I am also focusing more on what happens when, hopefully, I go beyond the end of the ruler.

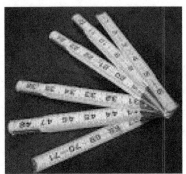

"Don't know if this makes much sense or is in any way applicable to your effort, but it seems to me your audience may benefit from an increased awareness of time and what they can do to productively live their lives now with that goal of having an enjoyable existence in the future."

That's a positive view. Here are two more, each with a different perspective.

In his book *The Experiment,* Ian Brown rebels against aging through his diary that he starts at age 60. As recounted by Gerard Helferich in a "Wall Street Journal" book review, "His journal is largely a protest against decline. His hearing is fading, along with his memory. His knees ache. His arches have fallen. His face sags, and a patch of hair over his forehead resembles 'a random stand of corn that somehow got planted away from the main field.' He has rosacea, age spots and a hemorrhoid. Though he and his friends still hike and ski, it's a case of 'ever-older men doing daring things, to prove we're still daring, and therefore not older.' Mostly Ian Brown regrets not taking more risks ... he is afraid that he hasn't lived up to his promise ... A friend reminds him that we spend the first half of our lives wishing we looked like someone else and the second half wishing we looked like our former selves."

Willard Spiegelman, on the other hand, who was in his early seventies when he wrote *Senior Moments,* may be, Helferich says, "closer to the end than Mr. Brown, [but] he doesn't betray dread or regret but a gentle, teasing acceptance. 'We come into the world alone, with a cry ... we exit alone, to confront the final eternal silence. The fun, all the pleasure and adventure, lies in between.' [The two books'] striking dissimilarities – in content and form but especially in attitude and voice – derive from the authors' varying views on life more than from their relative ages or their divergent attitudes about the end of life. Whether we are 60 or 70, or 80 or 90, how fiercely we rage against the coming of that good night depends above all on how we have embraced the sum of our days."

...

For most of recorded human history, lifespans did not change. Then beginning in the late 1800s, life length took major leaps up. Life expectancy doubled in the twentieth century. At the time of Lincoln, the average lifespan was 38 years; today it is about 81 (women) and 76 years (men).

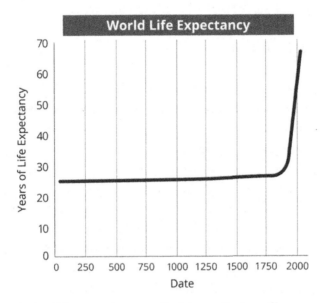

Why have lifespans increased? Most of the effect comes from decreased maternal mortality at childbirth from good obstetrical care, reduced infant mortality due to pre- and post-natal care, reduced childhood infection mortality due to vaccines, and greatly reduced deaths due to infections such as typhoid fever and tuberculosis as a result of safe water, clean sewers and pasteurization of milk. More recently, antibiotics are the prime example of an improvement that had a major impact on early mortality, as has care of those with trauma. In other words, deaths that used to occur in infants, children and young adults are largely curtailed today, with most deaths now occurring in only the older age groups and usually due to chronic illnesses—often related to a lifetime of adverse behaviors.

With fewer deaths in infancy, childhood and early adulthood, the age at death tends to cluster and looks like a waterfall when graphed. Most people begin to die near to the expected point, and then the drop-off occurs as the percentage of people still living declines precipitously. Fortunately, the early years of the "river" are a slow slope and the "waterfall" has been pushed downstream by years and decades, but eventually the time arrives.

Like a slow-moving river, we go through life in our twenties, forties and even sixties with little concern or thought about death. Then almost suddenly, we realize it is fast approaching. Can we as individuals push our personal waterfall further downstream? The answer is "yes," but to do so effectively requires starting back when we were not really thinking about it—as young adults or even better as children.

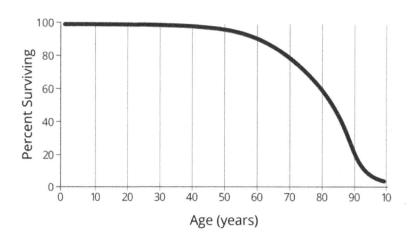

Longevity varies by location. Baltimore, Maryland, is a good example. For a person born in 2011, it is estimated by the Centers for Disease Control and Prevention that the average lifespan will be about 72 years. But the variability based on location within Baltimore of that birth is striking. A person, likely white and born in an affluent neighborhood, will live an average to 83 years. A child, likely black and born in a socially and economically distressed area, will die on average at age 63. Longevity varies by sex, race, location and many other factors, but in the end, it is only partly due to genetics, somewhat due to environment and very much due to how we treat our bodies over time. Of course, a person in a poor neighborhood has less access to healthy food, finds it unsafe to let the kids out to play, is chronically stressed just dealing with the bare necessities of life, and is barraged with advertisements for tobacco and alcohol while drug dealers abound on the corners and violent trauma is commonplace. In this case, it is not necessarily chosen behaviors but a lifestyle of necessity that determines variations in longevity.

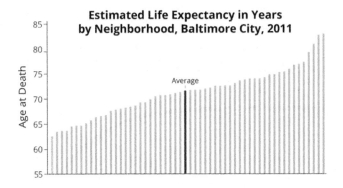

Essentially, the richest among us live the longest. Men who are among the richest 1 percent of Americans live until age 87 on average, but those in the bottom 1 percent live to about 72—a very marked difference. For women, the differences are 89 and 79 years, respectively. When graphed (see figure) the survival increases faster from poverty until about $50,000 per year and then continues to rise at a slower but quite noticeable rate. Of course, it is not money per se, but a combination of education, nutrition, trauma and lifestyle such as exercise, diet and smoking that impacts the length of life.[1]

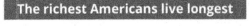

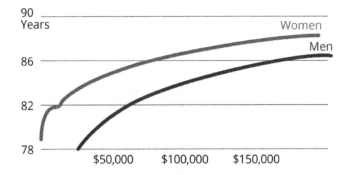

Between 1900 and now, there has been a truly immense change in the causes of death in the United States (the graphic below is a modification from the paper by Jones, et al.[2]). At that time, death came from typhoid, tuberculosis and pneumonia—all infections. Today, death is from heart disease, cancer, lung disease, stroke and complications of diabetes, high blood pressure, and obesity. Many diseases are increasing in numbers—Alzheimer's, Parkinson's and autoimmune diseases such as multiple sclerosis, diabetes type 1, Crohn's and celiac, rheumatoid arthritis and many others. These are chronic illnesses, meaning that once they develop, they don't go away. They are difficult to manage medically, and they are inherently expensive to treat. We can prevent or treat many infections today, which allows us to live long enough to develop one or more of these chronic illnesses. But does aging itself cause disease? Yes, but there is also a fundamentally marked change in how we live between then and now. In 1900, everyone was active all day, and food was local, fresh and simply prepared. Today, most people are sedentary, overweight and eat a diet high in calories and low in nutritional value. From farm and labor to an office desk, and from stay-at-home parents to the office as well. We are not moving. We are not eating fresh foods but instead prepared, processed and packaged foods with high concentrations of sugar, fat, salt and additives of truly questionable value. About 20 percent of us still smoke, and it seems that everyone is chronically stressed. Yes, smoking has declined substantially and that is good, but it has been superseded by a sedentary life of poor nutrition. Today, "sitting is the new smoking."

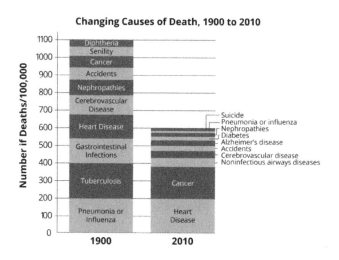

Changing Causes of Death, 1900 to 2010

It is instructive to look at not just the diseases present at death but the causes of those diseases that led to death. Study after study implicates the same lifestyle and behavioral factors—tobacco, diet, lack of exercise, alcohol abuse, drug abuse, trauma and sexually transmitted infections. The three most important are clear – tobacco, diet and exercise – to which I would add chronic stress and lack of a good night's sleep. The latter get all too little attention, but they are major contributors to aging and chronic illness development. (The chart below is based on a paper by McGinnis and Foege that addressed the antecedents to death-causing diseases in 1990)[3].

ACTUAL CAUSES OF DEATH IN THE UNITED STATES–1990	
Tobacco	400,000
Diet and Activity	300,000
Alcohol	100,000
Microbial Agents	90,000
Toxic Agents	60,000
Firearms	35,000
Sexual Behaviors	30,000
Motor Vehicles	25,000
Illicit Drugs	20,000

It is true that genetics plays a role in disease development, but it is a predisposition, not destiny. This is a very important concept. A predisposition is only manifested if something happens to "turn on" (express) that gene. These triggers are from the environment such as air pollution, but mostly they are the result of each individual's lifetime of behaviors. That is not to cast aspersion; rather it is to make the point that each of us needs to understand the impact of what we do or do not do each and every day and to make modifications where possible. The result will be not only health today but health tomorrow and for years to come with a longer life—one that may not be burdened with chronic illnesses.

Drs. Jones and Greene of Harvard and Hopkins, in an article about dementia commented: "The burden of disease in the 20th century, like that of the late 19th century, was not an inevitable fact of life, but a product of lives lived amid specific – and malleable – conditions."[4]

It is up to each of us to control those malleable conditions of our lives; it is possible, and the implication of doing so can be great. Despite genetic predispositions, abiding by a set of basic approaches to living can reap enormous benefits over the course of a lifetime. Yes, they require constant attention and can be difficult given the temptations from constant and aggressive marketers, but the result will be a longer life, a healthier life and a more fulfilled life.

CHAPTER TWO

NORMAL AGING: THE 1% PER YEAR LOSS

"If age is a thief, then the greatest treasure we lose is ourselves."—Michael B. Fossel[5]

Each day, each person grows older and, as everyone knows, a day will come when each person dies. Certainly, old parts wear out in the body just as in a car. But can anything be done to slow the process?

The percentage of the population that is "elderly" is rising fairly dramatically. In 1900, only 4 percent of the population was over 65 and only 1 percent over 75. By 1950, it was 8 percent and 3 percent, respectively. By 2000, it was 13 percent and 5 percent, now it's about 14 percent and 6 percent, and by 2030 will be 19 percent and 9 percent.

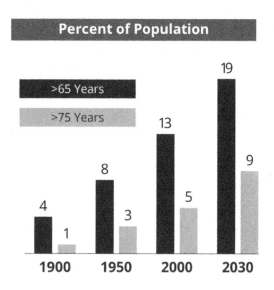

Percent of Population

>65 Years

>75 Years

| | 1900 | 1950 | 2000 | 2030 |

1900: 4, 1
1950: 8, 3
2000: 13, 5
2030: 19, 9

By 2030, it will be 19 percent and 9 percent.[6] More striking is the number of those over age 90, and even centenarians. Today the number of centenarians in the United States is just over 50,000, a 66 percent increase between 1980 and 2010, a period when the overall population of the U.S. grew by 36 percent.

There are many different concepts about aging, but for our purposes we'll consider aging gracefully or aging wisely. Most people would prefer to have a long life with the proviso that it is with good health while having some fun and enjoyment. That will be the theme of this book.

A story from a patient might give some perspective. Henry, a long-time friend of mine, called one day. He was in his seventies at the time, a widower, on Medicare and had multiple chronic illnesses. He told me that he was on 23(!) prescription medications and that not only was he feeling poorly, but they were much more expensive than he could afford to pay any longer—even though he had a Medicare Part D policy. He asked me what I could do to help. I told him I couldn't be his doctor at 400 miles away, but I could review the list of medications and give him some questions to ask his physician. It turned out that among his drugs were a couple for diabetes, a couple for heart failure, three for high blood pressure, one for cholesterol, one for depression, one for erectile dysfunction and one to reduce his prostate size.

I asked him about the high blood pressure medications. He said that every time he saw his doctor, they checked his blood pressure, found it to be about 150/85 and adjusted his medications. That seemed to be why he was on three drugs and at such high dosages. I asked him if he ever went to Wal-Mart or a drug store and measured his blood pressure there. Well, he said, "My son is an EMT and he comes by every Saturday to check up on me and he checks my blood pressure. It's always about 130/82, often a bit lower." I asked how long his blood pressure had been at that range, and he said, "Oh, it's been for five or six years at least. That's how long my son has been checking it." I asked, "When you go to see your doctor, what does he do?" He said, "Well, you know, I have four different doctors and each one checks my blood pressure and each one gets concerned because it is so high and when they do, they adjust my medications." The simple answer with Henry is that he really doesn't have high blood pressure as his regular pressures at home have demonstrated.[i] He has what is called "white coat" hypertension. In other words, any time he sees a health care professional he gets anxious and his blood pressure goes up.

But there is more to the story. He was getting a shot of testosterone once a month. I asked him what that was for. He told me it was because of impotence and his doctor thought this might help. It had not. I asked him about the drug to reduce his prostate size. He said that he had recently been in the hospital and had a serious infection that started in his urinary tract and went to his kidneys and then to his blood and then to his lungs. He had been in the intensive care unit, and, frankly, they saved his life. In the process, they decided he might have developed the infection because his prostate was large.

Let's take a look at his story. He was getting three drugs for high blood pressure that he probably didn't need. He then developed erectile dysfunction, and no one stopped to think about whether it was caused by the drugs, two of which are known to cause impotency. So he was given a shot of testosterone monthly, which may have increased the size of his prostate and in turn led to obstruction—and in turn led to an infection that almost killed him.

I suggested that what he really needed was a single physician as his primary care provider. After some hunting, he found an appropriate person and called me back a few months later to tell me he was now down to seven medications, feeling much better and certainly saving himself (and also his Medicare Part D insurance carrier) a lot of money.

There are some implications to Henry's story. Older individuals have multiple age-related impairments and they tend to have multiple chronic illnesses. As it turns out, the care of these illnesses is often not ideal. Maybe I should state this more forcefully: More often than not, chronic disease care is, well, less than ideal. And, of course, we know that health care costs are very high. One of the keys to changing this is really good comprehensive primary care, which Henry finally got. The other key is lifestyle modifications.

---

[i] The recent updates from the American College of Cardiology and the American Heart Association would consider 130/82 as hypertension stage 1. Normal now is less than 120 systolic and less than 80 diastolic. Less than 130/80 is classified as elevated blood pressure and 130-139/80-89 is hypertension stage 1. Many physicians would not treat an older person with Henry's level of blood pressure.

We'll deal with lifestyle in some detail as we go along and then return to primary care.

Old Parts Wear Out

As I mentioned earlier, just as a car ages, "old parts wear out." Most organ functions decline by about 1 percent per year. Of course, there is great variation. The decline varies from person to person and varies in the same person from year to year. But the 1 percent concept is a pretty good average to use for thinking and strategizing. This decline starts in earnest at about age 40, earlier in many cases (as described below) and continues throughout life. Fortunately, most of our organs have a huge redundancy, so we can afford these declines without any level of illness. But at some point, the decline reaches the point where we have a functional impairment that can be serious.

Hearing decline begins at about age 25 but is not noticed until much later. It is speeded by loud sounds – a rock concert, a jack hammer and loud music on iPods and MP3 players. Similarly, many people need reading glasses by age 40 even though they've had excellent vision for years; cataracts will occur later. Muscle strength and muscle size decline by age 50. Balance, not noticed until much later, starts its inevitable decline by then as well. Walking speed slows over time and endurance as well. What seemed like a trivial climb up a mountain trail now comes with shortness of breath and later seems nearly impossible. Meanwhile, internal organs such as the heart, lungs and kidneys slowly decline, as does brain function, especially cognition.

This normal aging process of old parts wearing out is universal and progressive. Let's use bone mineral density (BMD) as an example. BMD is a measure that is easily calculated to demonstrate the sturdiness of our bones. We start life with cartilage rather than bones, but as we grow as toddlers, then as children, then as teenagers, calcium, minerals and a protein collagen matrix make bones increasingly strong, reaching a peak around age 20. Once that age and that peak are reached, it can't go up any further—that's it. Then there is a plateau and around age 40, it starts to decline at 1 percent per year. At age 20, men's bone mineral density is, on average, higher than women's. Nevertheless, for women as for men, the decline is about 1 percent per year.

Menopause changes this; the rate of loss increases to perhaps 3 percent per year for a few years and then returns again to the 1 percent average decline.

There are three important points here. If we live long enough, our bone mineral density will decline to a level called osteoporosis, where a bone fracture becomes more likely if we fall. Since women start at a lower level and because they have an increased loss of bone mineral density during menopause, they reach that fracture threshold in life earlier than men. Since women tend to live longer than men, in total more women than men will have a fracture at some point in their lives. That is one of the risks of living longer.

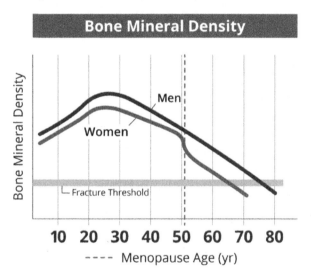

Cognitive function is another example; our brain loses some of its abilities as we age. This loss of cognitive function over time should not be confused with Alzheimer's disease. Nearly everyone who lives long enough will suffer from some cognitive decline, but only some individuals develop the disease known as Alzheimer's. As with BMD, we reach our peak cognitive function around age 20; it plateaus for about 5-10 years and then starts the slow decline. By age 50, we experience about a 4 percent loss of memory, reasoning and comprehension. By age 70, the loss is about 10 percent more. Given the great redundancy in our brains, it is not noticeable for some time. Eventually, we reach a functional threshold where our cognitive function begins to impair our ability. This becomes more apparent when an older person is engaged in highly technical activities, fast-paced activities, or in stressful situations (emotional, physical or health-related). Those challenges to cognition are less apparent when in highly familiar situations.

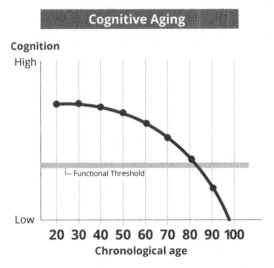

Our height drops over time. Most people lose about 1/32-1/16 inch per year beginning at age 40, so a six-foot man will be distinctly shorter at age 80. Muscle loss is another easily recognizable and measurable decline. As with bone strength, cognition, and height, muscles only slowly diminish in size and strength. However, the decline is definite, and during older years, the person will readily recognize that they don't have the strength that they used to have. It requires more exercise effort to maintain current muscle strength and mass. The medical term for significant muscle loss is sarcopenia.

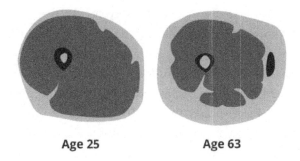

Age 25   Age 63

Our balance function declines as well. Balance depends on a combination of sight, vestibular (inner ear) function and the ability to sense where our joint positions are (proprioception). Each of these three diminishes as we age. Combine this with weakened muscles and bones, and the chance for a fall increases and the possibility of a fracture escalates since we depend on balance to not fall and on muscles to break a fall.

A few more comments on falls. According to the Centers for Disease Control and Prevention, almost 30 percent of older Americans fall per year and 38 percent of those reported a fall that limited activity or led to a doctor's visit. For those over age 65, falls were the most frequent cause of fatal and nonfatal injuries, with 27,000 deaths, 2.8 million ER visits, and 800,000 hospitalizations. Not surprisingly, the percentage of individuals that fell rose with increasing age, as did the percentage of falls that were serious. Healthy individuals of any age were less likely to fall or have significant injury than those with poor health (69 fall-related injuries per 1,000 compared to 480 per 1,000.) It is estimated that at least 25 percent of falls could be prevented by screening older adults for fall risk with gait and balance assessment, offering strength and balance exercises, managing medications known to be closely related to falls and, in many patients, prescribing added Vitamin D.[7]

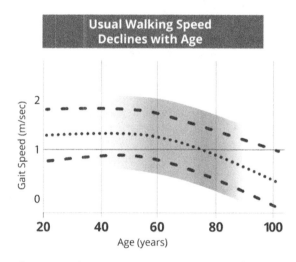

Usual walking speed is an interesting measure of aging impairments. We all know that as we get older, walking speed declines. Graphically, it starts at about age 60. It slowly starts to decline like other body functions and does so in a gradual but fairly steady rate. It turns out that mobility is actually a unifying concept in gerontology. Gait speed is adversely affected by aging impairments, chronic diseases, disuse, and deconditioning. Gait speed is a very powerful predictor of multiple adverse outcomes. It is actually a marker for "biological vitality." A simple test is to ask a person to walk at their usual pace along a distance of about 10 meters. This is timed for how long it takes to walk that distance. Any number of important outcomes can be associated with the gait performance test. As just one example, the number of deaths per hundred person-years is markedly up for those with a slow gait speed versus those with a rapid gait speed. The same can be said for admissions to nursing homes and for general well-being. (The two graphics are based on a lecture by Jack M. Guralnik, MD, PhD.)

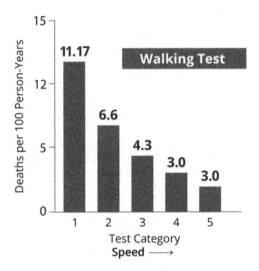

Do The Aging Processes Begin Early in Adulthood?

The answer seems to be yes. There is a fascinating study underway in the town of Dunedin, New Zealand. It began in 1972-73 when 1,037 individuals were enrolled to be followed from birth. By age 38, there was 95 percent retention of study individuals. The investigators, many from Duke University School of Medicine, evaluated them at age 26, 32 and 38 (and will continue to do so going forward) to determine if their biologic age would mirror their chrono-logic age or vary. They evaluated each participant using a measure developed by the National Health and Nutrition Survey (NHANES) that is known to predict later mortality. Their biologic age showed a typical bell-shaped curve relative to the chronologic age of 38 years. (The graphic is based on data from the paper by Belsky and others; see reference 8.) Notably, some participants were biologically as young as 28 and one as old as 61.

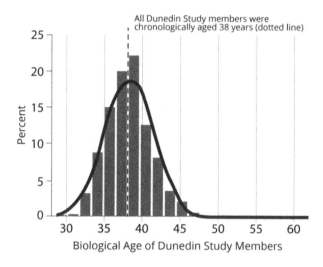

All Dunedin Study members were chronologically aged 38 years (dotted line)

Biological Age of Dunedin Study Members

They then analyzed the data obtained at ages 26, 32 and 38 from a set of 18 biomarkers known to be risk factors for various chronic illnesses such as HbA1c (a measure of blood glucose levels over prolonged time periods), waist-to-hip ratio (abdominal fat is dangerous), blood pressure, triglycerides, cholesterol, and body mass index (BMI). There was substantial variation among participants, with those that were biologically older having greater abnormalities in these measures. The biomarkers declined over the 12-year study period for all individuals. But declines occurred at varying rates among participants, with those that were biologically older showing the sharpest declines in function. Combining each of the 18 biomarker data points for each person over the three time points, the investigators calculated a "pace of aging" for each person. The pace of aging ranged from zero to 3 years of physiologic change for each chronologic year. In other words, some individu-als were aging much faster than their chronologic age would suggest.

They then asked the question, "Would these changes in biomarkers correlate with actual physical functions?" Those with more advanced biological age performed less well than their "younger" study members for the measures of balance, fine motor coordination and grip strength. They were also tested for cognitive function and were compared to the same testing done when they were children. Again, those with older biological age preformed less well. High resolution 2D photographs of the retina assessed the integrity of the vasculature as proxy for blood vessels within the brain. The biologically older individuals had narrower arterioles, which are associated with stroke risk, and they had wider venules, which are associated with dementia risk. Finally, they asked the participants to offer their own perceptions of their well-being, and via frontal facial photographs, asked a panel of students to assess the apparent age of each participant. Those with higher biologic age reported a perception of poorer health than did those of lower biologic age. The independent observers perceived those of higher biologic age as older than the others – yet they were all born during the same year.

It was notable that the study evidenced a systematic change in the 18 biomarkers known to relate to later (more often a few decades later in life) onset chronic illnesses. "Biological measures of study members' aging were mirrored in the functional status, brain health, self-awareness of their own physical well-being and their facial appearance. Study members who had older Biological Age and who experienced a fast Pace of Aging scored lower on tests of balance, strength, and motor coordination and reported more physical limitation. Study members who had an older Biological Age and who experienced a faster Pace of Aging also scored lower in IQ tests when they were age 38, showed actual decline in full scale IQ score from childhood to age 38 follow-up, and exhibited signs of elevated risk for stroke and for dementia measured from images of microvessels in their eyes ... it is possible to quantify individual differences in aging in young humans."[8]

Impairments versus Chronic Diseases

It may be useful to separate out what I will call impairments due to the aging process (that's the "old parts wear out concept") and age prevalent diseases. As to the impairments, as people age, they may have difficulty with their vision, hearing, mobility, cognition, memory, reflexes and balance. I think of these not as diseases but rather the effects of age.

The eye, for example, is at its peak function in the late twenties, including night vision, hand-eye coordination, depth perception, motion perception and color discrimination. But by the late thirties or early forties, it becomes difficult to focus on near objects because the ciliary muscle around the lens begins to weaken at the same time that the lens is becoming more rigid. Many people begin to have light sensitivity in their forties because the iris reflex response to light declines, allowing more light to enter the eye. I would label all of these as impairments that come with aging. Cataracts fall into this category as well, but retinal detachments due to diabetes would fall more into the realm of chronic illnesses.

On the other hand, chronic diseases such as heart failure, cancer, chronic lung disease, chronic kidney disease and diabetes occur more frequently as we age but are not necessarily due to age. That is an important concept. For example, coronary artery disease might lead to a heart attack in a man who is 67 years old, but that heart attack didn't occur in a vacuum just because of his age. The disease atherosclerosis really began in his teenage years or twenties, and slowly but surely plaque built up in his arteries until one of the arteries became sufficiently occluded and then impacted by local inflammation and plaque rupture that the heart attacked occurred at age 67. There is a similar situation with lung cancer. On average (and averages can be quite misleading because there is a very wide range around the average), tobacco-related lung cancer is diagnosed at age 72. But it didn't just develop then. If it was caused by smoking, then it began as a teenager when the person first sneaked one of his father's cigarettes and went out behind the garage for a smoke.

It has been said that aging is a bigger risk factor for these age-prevalent chronic diseases than all other causes combined, but I am not so certain. The prevalence increases dramatically with age (the graph shows that deaths from chronic illnesses and disability adjusted life year (DALYs) rises rapidly with increasing age, but is it the aging process itself that leads to chronic illness? It is not just aging but a lifetime of behaviors that have eventually culminated in diseases.

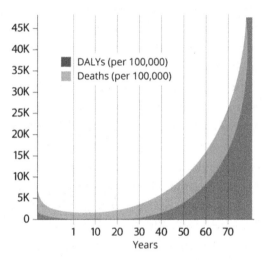

The "big four" adverse lifestyles are poor nutrition (and too much of it), lack of exercise, chronic stress, and tobacco. Add inadequate sleep, alcohol abuse, poor dental hygiene, drug abuse and driving impairments, including alcohol, drugs, and distractions such as texting. It is lifestyle behaviors that drive most chronic diseases – not all, of course – and, as a later chapter will detail, it is a change of lifestyle that can prevent perhaps 80 percent of the chronic illnesses that impact us as we age. That is an impressive reduction, so it is well worth understanding and appreciating the impact of lifestyle— both the positive and negative. After a discussion of some of the known physiologic impacts on aging, we will address how changing your lifestyle and environmental factors can have a positive impact on your health and lon- gevity. Although it would be best to start in childhood and early adulthood, *it is never too late to begin.* The effect will be nearly immediate and noticeable. Fewer chronic illnesses mean a healthier, longer life—certainly worth aim- ing for.

. . .

Note: I use the number 1 percent as a proxy for an inexorable continuing decline in organs and tissues. The exact number is highly variable from tis- sue to tissue, time to time, person to person. Think of it as a very rough average decline. Your genes have an impact but importantly, it is a decline that you can directly impact either positively or negatively with your life-style actions over time.

CHAPTER THREE

THE PHYSIOLOGY OF AGING

It is generally believed that age is the greatest risk factor for nearly every major cause of morbidity in the United States and other developed countries.

It might then follow that interventions that slow the aging process would have a greater effect on quality of life than disease-specific approaches. In other words, if aging could be slowed, then perhaps chronic illnesses would not occur. "Geroscience" postulates that biologic aging can be modifiable. If biologic aging is delayed, then the onset or progression of diseases that correlate with aging would be delayed as well.

This leads to an important concept that addressing aging, rather than specific illnesses may have broader implications for many diseases. This has been called the "longevity dividend."

Why is it that the human body (and all organisms) age? If we want to impact the aging process, it is critical to understand the cellular and molecular mechanisms that lead to aging. However, why we age is not known. Is there one fundamental reason? Or are there many that together drive the aging process and its timing? There are many studies underway to assess the aging process and why we age biologically. Interestingly, there is not a huge body of knowledge since grant funding agencies don't emphasize research on aging. Plus, the Food and Drug Administration doesn't look at aging as a disease, so it is not interested in pharmaceutical companies bringing them longevity drugs to evaluate. This has limited the industry's interest in research. These attitudes seem to be changing, but they help to explain why, despite all of today's biomedical knowledge, the aging process is definitely not well understood.

An obvious observation commented upon by Aristotle in about 350 BC is that larger animals tend to live longer than smaller ones, but the reasons – then and now – are completely unknown. Humans have been known to live to 122 years, but the average across the globe is about 71 years. In the U.S., lifespans today are about 77 years for men and 81 years for women. Those in the five Blue Zones (see Chapter 5) have a high proportion of individuals who live to be centenarians. These Blue Zones are in completely different parts of the world, and the individuals are of different ethnicities, religions, and food preferences, yet they are similar in living long lives. Why?

A recent review in the journal "Cell" attempted to integrate the knowledge of aging. Fundamentally, the authors argue that, "Several metabolic alterations accumulate over time along with a reduction in biological fitness." In other words, aging is about how cells' metabolism changes over time. Metabolism here refers to all of the myriad cellular activities that occur all of the time in each cell of the body. The authors indicate that there are various metabolic circuits that can be affected by genes, some that favor longevity and some that accelerate aging. They note that lifestyles, especially the "Western" hypercaloric diet and sedentary attitude have a detrimental impact on metabolic functions and thereby accelerate aging. Their concept is that steps to improve or promote metabolic "fitness" can extend lifespans.[9]

Here, in brief, are some of the developing scientific theories being investigated.

DNA Damage

The DNA in your cells is naturally damaged over time, but cellular mechanisms are capable of repairing the vast majority of lesions. Some nevertheless accumulate with age and eventually may include damage that impacts aging. Damaged DNA accumulates in tissues such as the brain, muscle, kidney and liver. Centenarians have high levels of innate repair capacity, often higher levels than individuals many decades younger.

DNA Winding: Tight Versus Loose

The double helix of DNA is normally "tightly" wound, but with aging it may "loosen." This impacts the expression of genes related to the aging process. Sirtuins, especially the enzyme SIRT1 (named from the word sirtuin and numbered for each type discovered), maintain the tight winding of DNA. But with age, the DNA winding loosens, leading to expression of genes that can cause cellular damage and ultimately lead to diseases. Some scientists strongly believe that this loosening of the DNA is the driver of aging. If so, enhancing the SIRT1 enzyme should lead to slowing aging or possibly even age reversal. Resveratrol, as found in low concentrations in red wine (see Chapter 9) in animal models lengthens life; it has beneficial effects by enhancing sirtuins. Although a pill sounds like a simple solution, on a current practicable level, it is known that a healthy diet and plenty of exercise will activate sirtuins.

Longevity Genes

Genes control cellular activity. Perhaps there are genes that either promote or diminish the opportunity for long life.

How do centenarians get there? In part, they had to avoid the problems of pregnancy, birth, early childhood infections, trauma during teen and early adulthood and then age-prevalent diseases such as cancer and heart disease in later life. Lifestyles are critical in this regard but not enough. Although genes are not fully understood, it is becoming clearer that some people are winners in the gene lottery and some are less fortunate. Some of the genes in question seem to be "protective" and impart a greater functional reserve to various organs and cellular metabolic pathways. Other genes are missing – ones that increase the risk for a specific disease. In addition, there may be genes that impact the "biologic clock(s)" that slow the aging process (see Chapter 4).

There is a study of some 600 long-lived Ashkenazi Jews between the ages of 95 and 112 in New York City. Some gene variants have been found in these individuals that tend not to be present in most others (and who do not live as long). Whether these represent genetic variations that help these particular individuals live a longer life is unclear. But they represent the beginning science that is trying to find reasons why some people live longer than others. There have been about a half dozen biochemical pathways and mechanisms recognized related to metabolism, growth, response to stress, stem cell viability, inflammation and proteostasis (or the "quality control" mechanism of the cell) that various researchers believe might have an impact on aging. Interestingly, these centenarians do not necessarily follow the "rules," as in, they do not necessarily eat a healthy diet, are overweight, don't exercise regularly, and smoke. In this case, their long lives are not lifestyle or environment-related but gene-related. Does that mean that there is no hope for the rest of us? Definitely not, as will be discussed ahead.

Based on studies of the roundworm *C. elegans* (a common organism used to study aging and various diseases), it appears that adult cells rather abruptly begin to age once reproduction has been initiated.[10] Conceptually, the organism understands that it has developed the means to reproduce and so can begin to age without preventing the continuation of its line. According to one of the investigators, R Morimoto, "All these … [metabolic] pathways that insure robustness of tissue function are essential for life, so it was unexpected that a genetic switch is literally thrown eight hours into adulthood, leading to repression … of the cell stress responses … This genetic switch gives us a target for future research."[11]

Overall, it appears that there are at least several dozen genes that impact aging negatively. Inactivating one or more can have a major impact on aging in animal models.

Telomeres

Telomeres are often described as the protective caps at the ends of chromosomes, like the ends of a shoelace. Composed of DNA like the rest of the chromosome, telomere function is unclear, but length variations are critical to cellular division and lifespan.

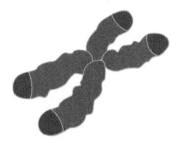

Telomeres shorten with each cell division and thus with age but need to be of a certain length for cells to continue to divide. Telomeres are measured in terms of DNA "base pairs," or the nucleosides or building blocks that make up the DNA strand. At conception, telomeres are about 15,000 base pairs long; at birth (after many cell divisions), they are down to about 10,000. They continue to decline at a rate of about 20-40+ base pairs per year. Once the length drops to about 5,000 base pairs, the cell can no longer divide and becomes senescent (see below) and ultimately dies. Does this shortening represent a built-in clock-like molecular aging mechanism? There is a normal enzyme in all cells called telomerase that can repair and lengthen telomeres. It is present in the embryonic, fetal and early childhood development phases but declines dramatically in mature cells and organs. Experiments to increase the amount of telomerase in the cells in some animal models have led to longer telomeres and longer lifespans. (Telomeres and telomerase will be discussed further in Chapter 10 .)

Stem cells

Stem cells are essential for life. Stem cells produce, for example, the constantly regenerating red and white blood cells of the blood stream and the lining of the intestinal tract whose cells turn over every few days. But with aging, their function is diminished. Exactly why is unclear.

Free Radical Damage to Cells

Free radicals can be produced by radiation that constantly impacts the Earth from space and from X-rays or products of nuclear bombs. However, most free radicals are a byproduct of normal cellular metabolism. A free radical is defined as an atom or molecule that has a single unpaired electron. Fundamentally, it means that the molecule is unstable and highly reactive. It "wants" to obtain the missing electron and will attempt to garner one from another molecule. The molecule that lost an electron is now the free radical and looks for an electron for itself. This creates a chain reaction wherein the very reactive free radical may damage a key biological compound or process. Cells have internal mechanisms to stop the chain reaction and render the free radical harmless using cellular antioxidants such as glutathione or nutritional antioxidants such as vitamins E and C. Generally, the cell can and will repair oxidative or free radical damage. But some damage may not be repaired, and sometimes this leads to significant cellular damage. Critical to this discussion is that certain types of damage to DNA can impact the aging process.

Mitochondria

Mitochondria are the energy factories of cells but can become damaged over time. Mitochondrial defects accumulate with age and have been created due to free radicals that are produced in the mitochondria. Free radical production appears to increase with aging and various chronic illnesses. An assumption has been that ingesting antioxidants would reduce free radical damage, but clinical trials have been unrewarding.

Rather than try to destroy the free radicals after they are produced, the more logical approach might be to shut down their production. Martin Brand Ph.D. and his colleagues at the Novartis Genomics Institute and the Buck Institute for Research on Aging screened 635,000 small molecules and found a few that would prevent mitochondrial free radical production. These have been quite effective in early laboratory studies of heart muscle and cultured brain cells.

But it may not be just free radicals that impact the mitochondria. Other research suggests that the changes in the mitochondria are due to DNA epigenetic changes (see below) that affect which genes are active and which are not.[12]

Heterochromatin

Heterochromatin is a tightly or densely packaged form of DNA. There is at least one gene that helps to stabilize heterochromatin through the expression of a protein of the same name.[ii] Damage to this gene creates cellular disorganization of the heterochromatin such that the DNA is no longer tightly packed together. This in turn effects whether genes are expressed by impacting epigenetic regulation (see below) of gene activity. It is believed that accumulated structural alternations in the heterochromatin may be a significant part of the aging mechanism.

Epigenetics

Epigenetics has to do with the chemical add-ons to DNA by methyl groups. These epigenetic changes can be created or modified by lifestyle activities (such as smoking, foods, exercise and stress) and they can be transmitted from generation to generation. Scientists are, therefore, looking at ways to affect epigenetics to our advantage and as a result possibly decrease age-prevalent chronic diseases. Epigenetic changes also serve as a biologic clock; see the next chapter.

Gut Microbiome

The gastrointestinal tract houses a diverse and extremely large number of bacteria, protozoa, viruses and fungi. They are known collectively as the gut microbiota, and their genomes are called the gut microbiome. Scientists have only begun to understand the microbiota in the past decade or so. Many, if not most, of the intestinal bacteria have never been successfully cultured, but with the advent of advanced genomic analysis, it has become possible to characterize them. There are about ten times more microbes (100 trillion) in our gut than all the cells of our body. The colon has the most, by far; the small intestines much less; and the stomach, which is acidic, holds relatively few bacteria. The colonic bacteria would weigh about one half pound or more and stool is composed of about 75 percent bacteria. They are an integral part of our lives and serve many important functions; it is a true symbiotic

---

[ii] The Werner syndrome RecQ helicase-like gene

relationship provided the microbiota are "normal." The microbiota maintains a barrier against the entry of harmful or pathogenic bacteria, help to synthesize some vitamins, degrade and ferment the fiber in foods to create an important nutrient for colonic lining cells, stimulate the immune system, and helps maintain the cellar integrity of the intestinal lining. Diet, exercise, stress and antibiotics lead to changes in its composition and it changes with aging. Those living in long-stay residential nursing facilities have a much different microbiota than those living independently despite similar ages. The microbiota of people in these long-stay facilities correlates well with age-related frailty but it is not clear which drives the other. The gut microbiota also correlates well with cardiac function, inflammation and innate immunity. Changes in the gut microbiota lead to changes in these functions, so it appears that it is the microbiota that are the driver, not the reverse. However, it is unclear if microbiota changes lead to the aging process or if the aging gut supports a changed microbiota. Perhaps both.

Among the useful compounds produced by the bacterial fermentation of fiber in the colon are acetate, propionate and butyrate. Acetate is used by muscles in the heart, kidney and brain as an energy source. Butyrate is a major energy source for colonic lining cells. It also increases the immune cells' anti-inflammatory effects, perhaps by its effect on macrophages to reduce production of inflammatory cytokines such as IL-6. (Cytokines are molecules produced by a cell of the immune system that communicates or signals other cells to an action. The cytokine IL-6 is one of the compounds that augment the production of the inflammatory response.)

Even normal bacteria produce substances that can be toxic to intestinal cells or the entire body if absorbed. Among these are the cell membranes of Gram negative bacteria, known as lipopolysaccharide (LPS.) LPS, also called endotoxin, causes inflammation. Constant exposure to LPS through a "leaky gut" results in systemic circulation of endotoxin followed by chronic inflammation in a variety of body locations. This, in turn, can lead to, among many other actions, anxiety and depression, heart and brain damage, muscle loss, and an acceleration of the aging process.

Dietary factors impact the gut microbiota. Fresh vegetables and fruits, high in fiber, are beneficial whereas simple sugars are deleterious and lead to inflammation. Think of it as feeding the "good guys" but starving the "bad guys" with high intake of fiber foods and low amounts of sugar. Unfortunately, the standard American diet (SAD, pun intended) does exactly the opposite. The fats in corn-fed meat are damaging whereas the omega 3 fatty acids of cold water fish are helpful. Indeed, the latter reduces inflammation.

Chronic inflammation is a major contributor to aging and age-prevalent chronic diseases. When colonic lining cells have insufficient butyrate from fiber fermentation by the microbiota, the lining cells lose their ability to prevent the entrance of inflammatory compounds such as LPS. When low levels of LPS continuously reach the systemic circulation, it produces chronic inflammation.

Specific approaches to slowing the aging process will be discussed later (Chapters 6-8,) but the above would make it obvious that a diet rich in fiber (such as fruits and vegetables, plus beans, lentils, and oats) would be beneficial whereas simple carbohydrates such as sugars and starches (as found in refined white flour in breads, pasta and pizza) that are rapidly digested, are of no value to the microbiota, and upset the normal balance, aiding the onset of inflammation. Ingestion of simple carbohydrates also augments the onset of obesity, metabolic syndrome and type 2 diabetes.

Consider an ongoing study on the island of Sardinia (one of the Blue Zones in Chapter 5) that involves 1,250 older people. Half will use the Mediterranean diet and half their standard diet. The study will evaluate how diet affects inflammation, the microbiota and various functional characteristics. But since these peoples tend to follow a Mediterranean-style diet anyway, it is somewhat unclear how effective the study will be in finding differences.

The microbiota are generally stable over long periods but can be altered by antibiotics and diet. Prebiotics are the digestion-resistant starches (fibers) noted above. Probiotics are bacteria that can be ingested orally, resist the acid of the stomach and help stabilize in a positive manner the normal microbiota. They usually do not colonize the gut, as in, they do not remain for any length of time, but they have a positive impact by inducing gene activity in the microbiota that reduces inflammation. Many fermented foods contain probiotic bacteria such as yogurt, kimchi, and sauerkraut. Probiotics are also available as capsules. No one really knows which bacteria are the most beneficial as probiotics, but based on current knowledge, the most common in commercially sold probiotic mixtures are Lactobacilli and the Bifidobacteria. [13]

Association studies (which are quite different from cause-and-effect studies) have linked the gut, oral and nasal microbiota with a variety of chronic illnesses. In sum, the microbiota may be critical to the aging process through their impact on the development of chronic illnesses, its production of low grade inflammation over long periods, and its impact on the immune system.[14] Although not proven, there is substantial association evidence that altering the microbiota may impact the aging process.

Long-lived Proteins

Some cells never divide in the heart and the brain, and some proteins in these cells are present throughout the life of a cell. Since they are not replaced on a continuous basis like other proteins, the question is whether these long-lived proteins are or can be damaged over time. It seems that they are in mice, especially in the brain, and this may have implications for aging. The long-lived proteins are part of the nuclear surface and have a control function as to what enters and exits the nucleus. As they degrade over time, they are not replaced and can allow toxins to enter, which in turn can damage the DNA and lead to aging.

Senescent Cells

Over time, cells have damage to their DNA. In many cells, this is quickly repaired while other cells die. And some cells become senescent or "retired." Although not active in the usual sense, senescent cells still produce a variety of cytokines that can be harmful to other cells. As the body ages, the number of senescent cells accumulates, and there is a theory that they are responsible for some or even most of the aging process. Darren Baker and Jan van Deursen, researchers at the Mayo School of Medicine, have studied these cells and found that they produce a protein called p16. When they inhibited a gene called BubR1 in mice, the mice accumulated senescent cells and began to age rapidly. When the researchers found a drug to destroy the p16 laden cells (the actual process was rather complicated), the mice improved. They still died earlier than normal, but they gained weight and were generally healthier.

Their next step was to study normal mice by administering the drug twice a week at middle age (again a complicated procedure) to destroy senescent cells. The mice lived an average 25 percent longer. Compared to those not treated, these mice lost less body fat as they aged, remained more active and had better heart and kidney function.[15] The researchers concluded, and many would agree, "Our proof-of-principle experiments demonstrate that therapeutic interventions to clear senescent cells or block their effects may represent an avenue for treating or delaying age-related diseases and improving healthy human lifespan."[16]

Not surprisingly, the company Unity Biotechnology, with van Deursen as a co-founder, was formed with venture backing in an attempt to make these observations clinically relevant. The company is evaluating a series of compounds that are particularly effective in destroying senescent cells. They have plans to attack osteoarthritis and glaucoma and perhaps later try to effect actual lifespan. According to the company's website, "We envision a future in which people get older without getting sicker—a future in which people stay healthy and mobile long into old age."[17]

As with other aspects reviewed here regarding the aging process, sound nutrition, regular exercise and stress reduction can all impact the production and destruction of senescent cells so they are less likely to accumulate over the years.

So far, it is clear that senescent cells accumulate with age and have an adverse impact on cell function. Their removal reverses damage to heart and kidney cells, reduces the development of cancer and might have an impact on survival.

. . .

There are many mechanisms involved in the aging process. Scientists have yet to identify which ones are most important, whether all are integral or whether some other(s) yet to be identified will prove most critical. But as more information comes to light, it is apparent that clinical trials seeking possible avenues for slowing the aging process and slowing the onset of age-prevalent diseases will markedly accelerate.

We all look forward to a long, healthy life; we would like to "age gracefully." But despite the intriguing studies presented here and in other chapters, the exact biological mechanisms of aging and its prevention are not known. This raises the question: Can we slow the aging process and prevent (or at least delay) the onset of the diseases that are so common in older years? The answer to both is "yes," but there is no Fountain of Youth or magic pill—yet. For now, it is all about lifestyle modification, including a sound diet, regular exercise, managing stress, getting a good night's sleep and no tobacco—preferably starting at an early age and sticking with it through the years.

Perhaps a bit of humor should end this chapter.

Jacob, age 92, and Rebecca, age 89, are excited about their decision to get married. They go for a stroll to discuss the wedding, and on the way, they pass a drugstore.

Jacob suggests they go in.

Jacob addresses the man behind the counter: "Are you the owner?"

The pharmacist answers, "Yes."

Jacob: "We're about to get married. Do you sell heart medication?"

Pharmacist: "Of course, we do."

Jacob: "How about medicine for circulation?"

Pharmacist: "All kinds."

Jacob: "Medicine for rheumatism?"

Pharmacist: "Definitely."

Jacob: "How about suppositories?"

Pharmacist: "You bet!"

Jacob: "Everything for heartburn and indigestion?"

Pharmacist: "We sure do."

Jacob: "You sell wheelchairs and walkers and canes?"

Pharmacist: "All speeds and sizes."

Jacob: "Adult diapers."

Pharmacist: "Sure."

Jacob: "We'd like to use this store as our Bridal Registry."[18]

CHAPTER FOUR

AN AGING BIOLOGIC CLOCK

Is there a biologic aging clock? If so, what is it, what winds it up, and what drives its timing?

There is indeed a clock – and maybe at least three clocks – built into our cells. One is the shortening of telomeres. The length of the telomere gives a rough estimate of age, particularly biologic age. It may or may not correlate closely with an individual's chronologic age, but its length does correlate with the approach of cellular and, ultimately, whole body death.

A second clock may be the accumulation of senescent cells. As they build up, the body ages due to their toxic byproducts. Scientists are studying whether a measure of their presence could be the equivalent to a biologic clock.

The third biologic clock, and the one most intensively studied to date, relates to epigenetics. New research shows that the number and placement of epigenetic changes correlate well with age. What is becoming clearer is that they correlate with cellular and whole-body demise as well. The particularly exciting notion is that epigenetics can be altered by what individuals do each and every day: nutrition, exercise, chronic stress, sleep.

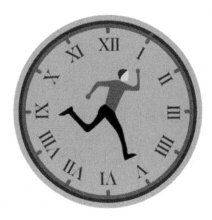

Steve Horvath, PhD, Sc.D., is a human geneticist and biostatistician professor at UCLA, where he has developed an algorithm based on epigenetics that measures the cellular biologic clock. His algorithm can closely estimate the age of the person from any cell. For example, white blood cells from a blood drawing are only a few days old at most, but their epigenetic pattern predicts very closely the chronological age of the person from which the blood was drawn.

Horvath expects that the most interesting use of the clock will be to detect "age acceleration," or the discrepancies between a person's epigenetic and chronological ages, either overall or in one particular part of their body (think back to the New Zealand studies in the last chapter).

Horvath and Dr. Brian Chen of the National Institute of Aging are evaluating 2,100 men and women ages 40-92 from the Framingham long-term heart study. They "concluded that for every five-year increase in age acceleration [meaning the epigenetic changes suggested a biologic age five years greater than the actual chronologic age], the risk of dying from any cause during the study jumped by 15 percent." From these and other studies, Horvath has shown that these epigenetic changes that demonstrate age acceleration correlate with earlier death. Still unknown is whether epigenetic age will specifically predict the onset of age-related diseases as opposed to overall mortality alone.

Horvath and Chen have collaborated with scientists from many countries to evaluate the DNA epigenetic changes from about 13,000 individuals and can now show that lifespan is shortened when the biologic age exceeds the chronologic age. Said differently, the epigenetic changes drive biologic aging and biologic aging correlates with death. At any age, a higher biologic age predicts a shorter lifespan, or a phenomenon they call age acceleration. Studies to date indicate that about 5 percent of the population ages at a faster biologic rate regardless of added risk factors such as gender or smoking, which means they will have a decidedly shorter lifespan. Horvath gives this example: "Two 60-year-old men, Peter and Joe, both smoke to deal with high stress. Peter's epigenetic aging rate ranks in the top 5 percent, while Joe's aging rate is average. The likelihood of Peter dying within the next 10 years is 75 percent compared to 60 percent for Joe."[19]

Horvath and Chen and their colleagues have looked at their data and adjusted them for various factors such as health status and known genetic factors. Clearly, their biologic age calculation predicts survival better than chronologic age. It appears that about 40 percent of the difference between chronologic age and biologic age is due to epigenetic changes that have been inherited, with the remainder of the epigenetic changes occurring during life. They conclude, "DNA methylation-derived [i.e., epigenetic changes] measures of accelerated aging are heritable traits that predict mortality independently of health status, lifestyle factors, and known genetic factors."

They continue, "The difference between DNA methylation age and chronological age predicts mortality risk over and above a combination of smoking, education, childhood IQ, social class, ApoE genotype [a known genetic risk factor for Alzheimer's disease], cardiovascular disease, high blood pressure, and diabetes. It may, therefore, be possible to think of DNA methylation predicted age as an 'epigenetic clock' that measures biological age and runs alongside, but not always in parallel with chronological age, and may inform life expectancy predictions. Our results imply that epigenetic marks, such as gene methylation, are like other complex traits: influenced by both genetic and environmental factors and associated with major health-related outcomes."[20]

Horvath's and others' studies raise this question: "Since the epigenetic methylation changes could be reversible, might it be possible to stop the progress of the clock and even turn it back?" To do so would require understanding what epigenetic changes are relevant to aging, isolating them and seeking ways to reverse the changes or block their expression.[21] That work is ongoing.

Meanwhile, as the suggestions of studies discussed in later chapters are invoked to slow or reverse aging, studying the epigenetic clock might give a reasonably rapid assay for effectiveness rather than waiting for years to learn if the intervention worked or not. As Horvath has said, "We don't have time, however, to follow a person for decades to test whether a new drug works. The epigenetic clock would allow scientists to quickly evaluate the effect of anti-aging therapies in only three years."[22] Although he mentioned drug therapies, it will also be equally, if not more interesting, to determine how sound nutrition, regular exercise, reduced stress, sound sleep and altered microbiota will impact these epigenetic changes—for the better. There is also substantial data that these lifestyle modifications can "undo" already present changes and prevent such changes into the future.

This is another example that genetics, including epigenetics, is not destiny. We can be still largely in control through how we live our lives. Meanwhile, it is clear there is a biologic clock, probably multiple, and further understanding them will lead to increased options to impact the aging process.

CHAPTER FIVE

THE BLUE ZONES: LESSONS FOR US ALL

As we touched on in Chapter 3, the Blue Zones are the five geographic regions of the world with the highest prevalence of people who are 100 or more years old. These Blue Zone centenarians don't just live longer than the rest of us—they also live healthier. They have lower rates of the common diseases that tend to reduce quality and length of life such as cancer, diabetes, heart disease and dementia. The five Blue Zones include the Nuoro Province of Sardinia, Italy; Okinawa, Japan; a community of Seventh-day Adventists in Loma Linda, California; the Nicoya Peninsula of Costa Rica, and Icarus, an island in Greece. Everyone can benefit from learning the secrets of the lifestyles of people in the Blue Zones.[23]

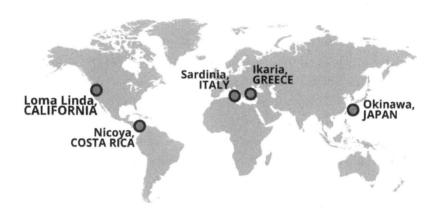

The Blue Zones studies began with the work of Gianni Pes, an Italian physician and statistician, and Michel Poulain, a Belgian demographer, who observed certain regions of the Sardinia Nuoro Province as having high numbers of centenarians.[24] Later, the National Geographic, the AARP, Dan Buettner, and the United Health Foundation teamed up to further study these areas.[25] Dan Buettner followed this with a bestselling book called *The Blue Zones*.[26]

The five Blue Zones are in many ways quite different. They are geographically spread across the globe, and the resident populations are genetically and ethnically different. Their religions are different, they live in dissimilar climates, and they eat different foods. Although there is no known scientific reason why residents of these five areas live a long time, they share certain overlapping characteristics that are known to be associated with good health.

First, Blue Zoners put family ahead of all other concerns. It is common for several generations to live together under one roof. Second, they take care of their bodies. Residents smoke relatively little and, although the diet is different by region, they consume a plant-focused, locally-sourced diet that includes plenty of vegetables and minimal sugar. Processed foods are uncommon, and most meals are made from scratch using fresh, local ingredients. Alcohol, usually wine, is consumed in moderation. In addition, people tend to eat meals together as a family or as a group, enjoying both the food and the company. Eating on the run is very rare. Also, physical activity is important. Residents engage in constant moderate physical activity throughout the day along with and as part of an active lifestyle. Fifth, residents of these zones participate in a high level of social engagement with their friends and family relative to other regions. Sixth, the elderly are included in the community. As individuals and as groups, they can be described as being physically and mentally active throughout their lives. The elderly continue to be active and contributing members in their families and communities.

In Okinawa, Japan, for example, an isolated island to the south of the Japanese mainland, individuals know their neighbors, are supportive of each other and have a strong sense of community spirit. Everyone is physically active; it's an integral part of living. Exercise does not occur in the gym but as part of everyday life, which includes the elderly as well. Older individuals continue to do their work as they always have. There are few cars and many people walk to the store, work, and friends' houses. They live naturally in their environment. Elders are respected and believed to have a true value to the community. There is a strong belief that life has a purpose. Each person has a strong sense of meaning in life and a reason to get up in the morning. Locals call this "Ikigai," which is a combination of the words "life" and "value." For an elderly Okinawan, this might be something as simple as working in the herb garden outside the kitchen door, participating in a hobby, or spending time with family. The core belief is in a purpose and meaning to life.

Okinawans eat a local plant-focused diet. As Okinawa is an island, there is a high consumption of seafood, both fish and shellfish, as well as sea vegetables. Staples of the diet include a purple sweet potato unique to the region. They also eat local fruits and vegetables and drink an anti-inflammatory fermented turmeric tea (more on the connection between inflammation and longevity in a later chapter). Processed and packaged foods are uncommon and sugar consumption is low. Similarly, the Nicoya Peninsula of Costa Rica is geographically isolated from the rest of the country, and the Nicoyan lifestyle is like the one on Okinawa. They have a high level of daily physical activity that they maintain into old age. Families are tight knit, with many generations living together under one roof. Residents eat "real food," not prepared, packaged or processed foods. The most common foods are rice and black beans plus fruit, cheese, eggs and corn tortillas with nearly every meal. Compared to other Blue Zones, in addition to locally caught fish, Nicoyans eat most meats, including chicken, pork and beef, which is all grass-fed, never grain-fed in feed lots. They also eat most fruits. Anecdotally, my daughter traveled to Nicoya a few years ago and noted that the food was fresh, local, and simply prepared. She was also impressed by the Costa Rican spirit of "Pura Vida," which is Spanish for "Pure Life." It reflects a fundamental optimism toward life.

As we can see from these notions of Ikigai and Pura Vida, individuals on both the Costa Rican Nicoya Peninsula and on Okinawa have a high level of thankfulness—gratitude for life and what life brings. Their stress seems to be low, and they accept whatever comes along. There is a strong sense of resilience and they "shrug off" adversity without holding personal grudges, which is an important component to low stress. We'll talk about this important characteristic of the Blue Zones and give specific techniques to develop gratitude and thankfulness as part of an overall stress management strategy in a later chapter.

My wife and I think of her Uncle John as embodying many of these attributes. He saw life as fundamentally positive, good – with its ups and major downs to be sure – but good nevertheless. He was resilient, able to get past adversity, never held a grudge and had a sense of everyday thankfulness.

Sardinia and Icarus residents follow similar patterns. They follow the classic Mediterranean diet, more or less. I point this out for those readers who think they don't want to eat nor have access to, the foods of Okinawa, are not particularly interested in the beans and rice culture of Costa Rica, and don't want to be vegetarians. Most Americans can relate to the Mediterranean diet with its great variety of foods. The keys are to keep added sugar to an absolute minimum, reduce meat consumption, eat a broad variety of vegetables and fruits, consume only whole grains (not refined white flour or white rice), and add in nuts and seeds. Olive oil is the one to use for salads and cooking and enjoy some wine.

Loma Linda is different from the other Blue Zones in that it is a relatively recent community that includes individuals and families of various ethnic backgrounds rather than centuries-old, ethnically-homogeneous communities. Brought together by their faith that the body is a temple and should be respected, they eat a semi-vegetarian diet that includes little meat but lots of vegetables, fruits, nuts and seeds. There are a few fast food restaurants, but eating there is an occasion, not a regular occurrence. They do not smoke or drink alcohol. They are active. Their faith and church help them remain calm in the face of life's challenges. Most attend church services regularly and engage in many of the community-church social activities.

In four out of five Blue Zones, the exception being Loma Linda, healthcare is relatively limited compared to what Americans would normally expect. It's pretty much primary care only with medical centers far away and hard to access. Yet their health is good, and their prevalence of chronic illnesses is much lower than what is found in the United States.

In Acciaroli, Italy, a town near Naples, lifespans are long. One of every 163 Americans is above the age of 90, according to the 2010 U.S. Census. But in Acciaroli, about one in 60 is over the age of 90. As with people living in the Blue Zones, these residents have few of the impairments of aging described in Chapter 2 such as cataracts. They also have a relatively low incidence of the age-prevalent diseases such as cancer, heart disease and Alzheimer's disease. Of course, there may be some genetic factors that have a significant impact in this relatively close-knit community. But aside from genetics, the absence of a more "modern" diet with its processed foods, added sugar and salt and high intake of sugary drinks is striking. In that sense, they are certainly not "modern." The residents credit the local rosemary plant. It's quite strong smelling and is used every day as part of meal preparation. Perhaps it is the rosemary but perhaps it's that they follow a Mediterranean style diet, they are outside and walking all the time, they manage stress well and they are very interactive with each other. [27]

Loma Linda University is conducting a long-term study of some 96,000 Adventists from across the US and Canada.[28] Some preliminary findings are: Those that follow a vegetarian diet (semi-vegetarian, pesco-vegetarian, lacto-ovo–vegetarian, or vegan) tend to be substantially less heavy than their non-vegetarian counterparts. Cholesterol is lower, blood pressure is lower, diabetes type 2 is less common as is the metabolic syndrome. The differences have a gradient – the stricter the vegetarian diet consumed correlates with a lower level of each measurement. All-cause mortality was also less.[29] These are impressive findings. They do not prove causation, but the observations are striking. It is also important to note that diet was not the only element that differentiated them from others. They tended to watch less television, slept longer, ate more vegetables and fruits and ate more beans and nuts. The study will also evaluate, over time, the impact of stress, exercise, social engagement and faith.

Recall from an earlier chapter that the number and percentage of older individuals is rapidly escalating. Americans are living close to twice as long now (78 years) as they did in 1900 (47 years) or an amazing increase of about 30+ years. However, it is worth looking into the numbers. It does not mean that most people actually died at age 47. The average includes those who died in infancy and of childhood infectious diseases, teenage and young adult trauma, complications of childbirth and those who lived for many decades such as our Founding Fathers—George Washington, Thomas Jefferson,

Benjamin Franklin and John Adams. It was an average of all of these. Infant mortality today is much less than in 1900 and maternal mortality is rare. Vaccines prevent most of the childhood infectious deaths, and good trauma care saves the lives of many young adults. Although some young adults still die young, not nearly as many die as in the past, and some of medicine's advances are helping those with chronic illnesses to survive for extra years. We can expect that the average age of death will further increase with better public health and medical care. However, the recent rapid rise of obesity and the metabolic syndrome with subsequent diabetes, cancer, stroke, kidney failure, and heart disease is of great concern. All of these diseases are chronic and are directly related to diet, exercise and stress.

Throughout this book, I will be recommending a plant-focused diet heavy in vegetables, fruits, nuts, seeds and whole grains, fish, some dairy products, limited meat and as little sugar as possible. It's best to avoid prepared, packaged, and processed industrialized foods and make meals an event with friends and family. I also recommend walking at least 30 minutes a day for five or six days a week. The people in the Blue Zones eat this diet normally and walk regularly. They don't make a particular time of day for walks. Instead, good food and walking all the time is part of their life. Because these regions are isolated, they simply didn't have stores with many processed or prepared foods and very few fast food outlets. This was true for those over 100 years of age, but much has changed in terms of diet and habits. The younger generation often lives differently, and their lifespans are shortening—Okinawa now has a lower lifespan than the rest of Japan.

In the last century, we have moved away from a sensible, healthy diet, and daily physical activity. We're fortunate to have all sorts of labor-saving devices such as washing machines, dishwashers, cars, and bicycles, and it is certainly easier to pick up carry out or order in pizza or to stop at the nearby fast-foot restaurant. But these have kept us from the quality meals and constant daily activity that was so valuable for our ancestors and which is so valuable for individuals in the five Blue Zones. That's not to say they don't have labor-saving devices or never eat out, but they select good foods that are simply prepared with minimal added fat, sugar, and salt and they are constantly active and on the move. They also seem to know how to control the stresses of everyday life or at least let them "run off their backs." What we as a society need to do is take time away from work, computers, iPhones and iPads, and get out into the community and do so with our feet.

Briefly summarized, the residents of these Blue Zones and Acciaroli, Italy, engage in moderate regular physical activity, have a moderate calorie intake that is largely plant-based, eat fresh foods prepared from scratch with limited processed or packaged foods, have a sense of life's purpose and have a remarkable facility for stress reduction. They drink alcohol in moderation, mostly wine, and they especially have a close-knit community spirit and engagement.

These are lessons everyone cannot only contemplate, but seek to emulate. These lessons are quite different from how most Americans live their lives today; it is time for a change. Such a change will certainly reap huge benefits going forward in life.

If it is not yet clear, here are some specific suggestions that you can follow. Each will be elaborated upon in the following chapters.

- Eat real, locally-sourced food, organic if possible, with a heavy emphasis on multiple, colorful vegetables. Specifically, cover two-thirds of your plate with vegetables and add a good helping each day of fresh (or frozen but not canned) fruits. Eat whole grains—not products made from refined white flour such as most breads, pies, cereals, cakes, cookies, pasta and pizza crusts. Include nuts and seeds plus olive oil for cooking and salad dressings. Eat fish in abundance, especially fin fish. Limit meat to a few times per week, and focus on grass-fed, not grain-fed sources. Consume sugar sparingly, which means avoiding sodas, candy and many processed foods such as most cereals.

- Move your body. Not just for 30 minutes at some predetermined time, although that is important, but move throughout the day. Include resistance exercises. This does not need to be at the gym. It could be walking around the block, or it could be gardening. Choose to take the stairs instead of the elevator. Walk instead of drive.

- Manage your stress. Include meditation each day or yoga a few times per week. Throughout the day, stop and take a few deep breaths. Look around. Enjoy. Be grateful for what you have.

- No tobacco.

- Get a good night's sleep.
- Stimulate your brain. It's fun to do and will reap big rewards. Be social: make, keep and interact with your friends.
- Give consideration to your life's purpose. You have a purpose and a direction though you may not know what it is. You can find it in the quiet of meditation. When you find it, you will realize it. Trust the signals that come to you. Think about your life's purpose. You may never have given this much thought before. Now would be a good time to start.
- Surround yourself with community. What does this mean? Find the people who are supportive and a positive influence in your life. This may be your family, your friends, or your neighbors. Create opportunities to spend time together.
- Find ways to get involved in your community. Studies have shown that people who volunteer to help others are happier and have higher levels of gratitude and thankfulness.

These are challenging recommendations, but certainly not impossible. Take it in steps. Be proud of what you accomplish, not annoyed at what you have not done. Then do more tomorrow and next week.

We'll go over each of these recommendations in more detail in the following chapters.

CHAPTER SIX

SLOWING AGING WITH LIFESTYLE MODIFICATIONS

Can we slow the aging process? The answer is a definite "yes." It's not easy and requires some real diligence, but nevertheless, aging can be slowed.

It would be useful to start with a quiz—the answer to which may be a surprise. It certainly was to me. Here is a list of five well-accepted healthy behaviors. The question is, what percent of Americans can answer "yes" to all five questions?

1. Exercise 20 minutes three times per week.
2. Do not smoke.
3. Eat fruits and vegetables regularly.
4. Wear seat belts regularly.
5. Have an appropriate BMI (the ratio of height to weight).

Here is a clue to the answer: We know that 20 percent of Americans smoke, which means the highest number who could answer "yes" to all five would be 80 percent. Also note that the five behaviors are not written in a very quantitative manner. For example, it says "eat fruits and vegetables regularly," but it does not say how many servings and what regularly means. Exercising 20 minutes three times a week is clear, but it does not say what type of exercise; it could be strenuous, or it could be just walking. Still, with these five and the fashion in which they are written, what percent of Americans can say "yes" to all five?

The answer, disappointingly, is only 3 percent. Three percent is a remarkably poor showing for our society!

The goals of preventive aging should be threefold. First is to prevent an acceleration of the normal aging process and even to slow it down. The second is to prevent age-prevalent diseases such as heart failure, cancer, Alzheimer's, various autoimmune diseases, and chronic lung disease from ever occurring. The third is to diagnose early and treat immediately whenever one of these diseases does occur.

As I mentioned previously, we all know "old parts wear out." It is equally true for the human body. But less appreciated is the fact that we can either slow or speed up the process, just as good preventive maintenance and careful attention can keep a car running for a long time while abusive driving and little attention will lead to wear and tear of the car at a fast clip.

The first graphic depicts a decrement of 1 percent per year in function of any organ. The graph begins at age 20 with the decline beginning at age 40 and the graph is set up to end at age 100.

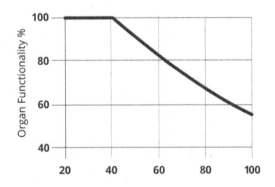

The next graphic includes what would happen if one could speed the functional decrement to 1.25 percent or if one could slow it to 0.75 percent. As in the previous graph, the decline is set to start at age 40 and continues on to age 100. It is clear from the graph that if we increase it by just 0.25 percent per year to 1.25 percent, at the end of the 60 years there is quite a marked added loss of function. On the other hand, if one slows it down to 0.75 percent per year, there is a rather dramatic reduction in the functional loss over time.

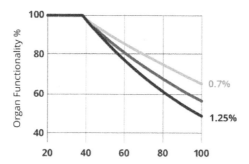

If one started the decline from the average 1 percent to 0.75 percent at age 60, would that still have an impact? The answer is yes – not as striking as if one started at age 40 – but still a very definite impact. It is clear that a program that slows the aging process by just 0.25 percent per year will have a significant and useful effect. Starting it early in life will have an impact similar to compounding interest—it just gets better and better to your advantage over time based on when you start.

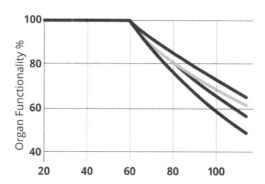

There is another important point though. The higher the level one starts at, or said differently, the greater the function of one's organ of interest at age 40, then the longer it will take to reach a functional level that compromises health and wellness.

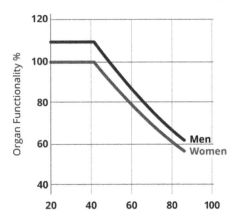

Let's return to the three examples of functional loss (bone strength, cognition, and muscle mass and strength), each losing about 1 percent per year beginning in early adulthood.

Reminder: As stated earlier, I am using 1 percent as a proxy for a decline that varies from person to person, time to time, and organ to organ. The range is wide but the concept of continued decline, a decline that can be altered with lifestyle modifications, is the critical point.

Bone Strength

Recall that bones gain in strength until about the age of 20, then it plateaus until about the age of 40 and begins that slow 1 percent decline for the rest of life. Women in general do not reach the same peak level of bone mineral density as men and, given that lower level and the speed up for a few years at menopause, they reach the fracture threshold sooner than men. Consider the graphics again, and it is clear that slowing that process in either men or women by 0.25 percent per year will have a huge impact in later life as to whether or not there is likelihood for a bone fracture. It is therefore important for our grandsons—and especially our granddaughters—to start out at an advantage. Getting them to eat a healthy diet and exercise aggressively as children and as teenagers will mean they will start out adult life with a higher absolute level of bone mineral density from which they will then decline. But how do they slow the decline once it starts?

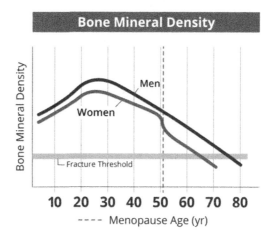

There are a number of adverse factors that can speed up the loss of bone mineral density. Among them is chronic stress. Protective factors include being physically active and eating a good diet throughout life. It is never too late to begin a good preventive maintenance program, so it is never too late to become physically active, eat a more nutritious diet, and deal with chronic stress.

Bone Mineral Density	
Adverse Factors	**Protective Factors**
• Low BMD at Age 20	• Physically Active
• Chronic Stress	• Good Nutrition

Cognition

The same issues apply to cognitive aging. If one challenges the brain at a young age so that by the beginning of adulthood your brain or cognitive function is at as great a peak as possible, then you are at a higher level before it begins to decline over the course of adult life.

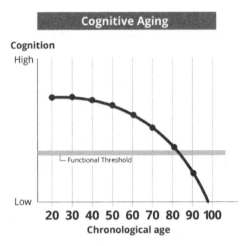

There are a number of factors that speed up the process of cognitive aging, and these include vascular conditions, chronic stress and metabolic syndrome (defined as three of these five: waist circumference over 40 inches for men or 35 inches for women, blood pressure over 130/85mm Hg, HDL {i.e., "good" cholesterol} below 40mg/dl, triglycerides greater than 150mg/dl, and blood sugar elevated over 100mg/dl).

On the other hand, there are protective factors against cognitive aging, including being physically active, having good nutrition, being intellectually challenged and stimulated and being socially engaged. It might be a surprise that physical activity is important for brain function, but multiple studies have demonstrated that this is extremely important. It may not be a surprise that good nutrition makes a difference and that there are certain foods that are particularly important, especially among the fruits and vegetables. Likewise, there are foods that have a negative effect, including sugar. Especially important in older individuals is to remain intellectually challenged and socially engaged. There is substantial information, although perhaps not strong proof, that intellectual challenge, such as playing chess or bridge or being involved in a study group that requires interchange with other people, is advantageous. Sitting in front of the television set or reading a book really doesn't constitute intellectual challenge, but if that book is discussed in a book club where each person has to defend their thoughts and positions, that becomes an intellectual challenge. Social engagement is equally important for older individuals. Those who become reclusive because of disease or an inability to get to locations where they can interact with others face a cognitive aging rate increase.

Cognitive Aging	
Adverse Factors	Protective Factors
• Vascular Conditions	• Physically Active
• Metabolic Syndrome	• Good Nutrition
• Chronic Stress	• Intellectually Challenged

Be curious. Do different mental activities rather than the "same old, same old." Blend mental activities with physical activities. For example, learning a new dance step requires "thinking" by paying attention to the music, getting the steps correct, moving at the same time, and being socially engaged. Playing a musical instrument is both a mental and physical activity that ties, for example, finger movements with musical patterns in the brain. Learning a new language is a good mental exercise, and meeting with a group of co-learners forces one to use these new abilities.

Neuroscientists call the brain "plastic," meaning that it can be strengthened with use just as your muscles can.

Muscle Mass and Strength

Here is an aphorism which I find very relevant: "Sitting is the new smoking." The point is that there has been enormous progress in reducing the number of individuals who smoke over the last couple of decades, and that has had a very profound positive impact in lowering the rates of heart disease, lung disease and lung cancer. But at the same time, there has been a great increase in the number of people who are couch potatoes.

Sarcopenia is the developing loss of muscle mass and strength that comes with aging (and some diseases). It means not just less strength but also reduced metabolism, greater likelihood of falling and an inability to do general activities of daily living. It is critical to maintain muscle mass and strength, which means regular aerobic and weight-bearing exercises. Strong muscles help you get around and protect you if you fall. The combination of weak muscles, impaired balance and osteoporosis leads to bone fractures during falls.

Some studies have shown that people lose about 30 percent of their muscle mass and strength between ages 50 and 70, a rate greater than the usual 1 percent per year. But research has also shown that mass and strength can be slowed considerably with exercise. Exercise positively affects tendons and bone. Although moderate exercise is fine, greater intensity for short durations is better, noted elsewhere as High Intensity Interval Training (HIIT.) For example, when riding an exercise bike in the gym, pedal at a comfortable rate for five minutes to warm up but then push it to your maximal level for 30 seconds. Slow down for 90 seconds to recuperate and then speed up again to your max for 30 seconds, slow down for 90 seconds and continue repeating for about 8 cycles. Do this twice per week. Initially you probably cannot go 8 cycles but with repeated practice your tolerance with go up.

Muscles are meant to be used, otherwise it leads to a loss of muscle mass as one ages. The graphic below shows a cross section of the muscles in the leg in two groups – those who exercise and those who do not. The difference is striking and should be a wake-up call to anyone who does not do both aerobic and resistance exercises regularly.

Preventing Age-Prevalent Disease

The leading causes of death in the elderly are heart disease, cancer and stroke—no surprise here. Each of these is largely, but not entirely, preventable by attending to your lifestyle. Unfortunately, most Americans eat a non-nutritious diet and too much of it, don't get enough exercise, are chronically stressed and 20 percent smoke. The result is a population that is obese with high blood pressure, which has led to a developing epidemic of diabetes and will lead to a high incidence of heart disease, cancer and stroke. It behooves everyone to address personal lifestyle changes, beginning at whatever age one may be today and following through over the years. It is never too late to begin. Many other chronic diseases, especially autoimmune diseases, are also negatively impacted by adverse lifestyles; it is worth changing course now.

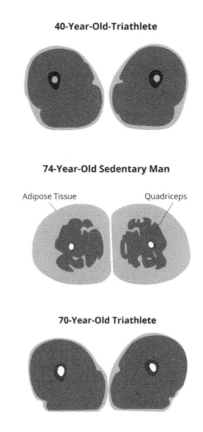

40-Year-Old-Triathlete

74-Year-Old Sedentary Man

Adipose Tissue   Quadriceps

70-Year-Old Triathlete

Cross section of muscles from Buck Institute.
Compliments of Frank Jannotta, PT

Various studies have aptly proven this contention. For example, in one study with long-term follow-up, it was found that those without diabetes, hypertension or obesity at age 45 lived 11 (men) or 15 (women) more years without heart failure compared to the age of onset of heart failure for those who had these diseases. Avoiding three risk factors (hypertension, obesity and diabetes) decreased later life heart failure by 86 percent. Clearly, these are issues to address in one's lifestyle considerations.

A study reported in the "New England Journal of Medicine"[30] that looked at a large number of individuals over many years dramatically makes the point. The researchers evaluated genetic data, adherence to a healthy lifestyle and onset of coronary artery disease from four large cohorts that totaled 55,000 individuals followed for many years. Not surprisingly, those with the highest genetic risk had nearly twice the incidence of coronary events than did those in the lowest genetic risk group. Those who maintained a healthy lifestyle (defined as not smoking, not obese, engaged in regular exercise and ate a healthy diet) had a much lower risk of coronary disease than those who were not so inclined. None of that might seem intuitively surprising, but importantly, even those with the highest genetic risk of heart disease (graphic below) reduced their relative risk by nearly 50 percent by adhering to at least three of the four healthy lifestyle factors.

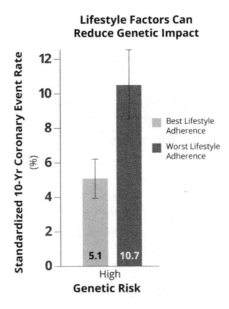

Of course, *slowing* aging does not equal *stopping* aging. Each year we get older. Diseases still can and will occur. But slower aging and fewer chronic illnesses beats the alternative.

SUMMARY

- **Slow Physical Decline & Onset of Chronic Illnesses**

  –Exercise, Sleep, Diet, Stress, Tobacco

- **Slow Cognitive Decline**

  –Physically Active
  –Intellectually Challenged
  –Socially Engaged

Investing in health is like any type of investing—it compounds over time. The best time to start is as a child or a young adult. If you are a grandparent, now is the time to help your grandchildren begin good habits of lifestyle. Remember that starting anytime pays a dividend, so get started even if you are far along the path of life. It is never too late to start. We are living longer, so let's live healthier.

CHAPTER SEVEN

SPECIFICS OF LIFESTYLE MODIFICATIONS

The basic steps of preventive aging are really one in number: lifestyle modification. Modifying lifestyle can be difficult, no question about it, but it is critical. There are a number of steps that are essential. Again, avoid tobacco, and if you smoke, it is never too late to quit. Reduce chronic stress. Eat a nutritious diet. Engage in physical exercise on a regular basis. Get a good night's sleep. Add to these intellectual stimulation and social engagement to maintain cognitive function. And then remember the importance of good dental hygiene, keeping vaccinations up to date, safe driving, dealing with loneliness and finding fulfillment.

These are not necessarily easy to achieve, but they are very important. Each will be discussed in more detail. It is also important to follow your doctor's advice about reducing elevated blood pressure, reducing elevated cholesterol (low density lipoprotein or LDL, the "bad" cholesterol) and maintaining a normal level of blood sugar. Lifestyle modifications may be enough to bring these into normalcy, but if not, your doctor may prescribe medications. Also, don't forget to get your annual flu shot and keep your vaccines up-to-date—if you are over 60, then shingles (it is not clear how often if at all this should be repeated), pneumonia every five years, and tetanus and diphtheria (Td vaccine) every 10 years; the combined Tdap for tetanus, diphtheria and pertussis as one of these boosters if not obtained earlier in life.

Experts are certain that this combination of lifestyle modifications, along with medical interventions as necessary, will reduce the risk of chronic illnesses by more than 80 percent. Now that is significant and makes the effort worthwhile.

Steps of Preventive Aging
• Lifestyle Modification
• Lifestyle Modification
• Lifestyle Modification
IT'S HARD BUT CRITICAL There is No Pill - No Foundation of Youth

Nutrition and Diet

"If we could give every individual the right amount of nourishment and exercise – not too much and not too little – we would have found the safest way to wealth."—Hippocrates.

That was 2,400 years ago, and it is still the best advice.

The aim should not be "weight loss" or "dieting." Rather, the aim is to modify behaviors or lifestyle. That is the goal. If lifestyles are changed to include appropriate eating patterns and appropriate food intake, along with exercise and less stress, then the weight loss will occur. Just dieting to remove weight is never permanent because once the weight is off, the old patterns return, along with the weight. The goal is health, not a specific weight.

A good place to begin is to understand and follow the Mediterranean diet. It consists of extensive fresh vegetables and fruit each day, plus regular servings of nuts, seeds, beans and whole grains such as whole wheat, oats and brown rice. Don't forget olive oil and fish with a glass of wine but limited meat and very little added sugar. This is widely considered to be a sound, healthy diet. As a general rule, the food is prepared "from scratch" in the kitchen, not processed from manufacturers or prepared from the corner deli.

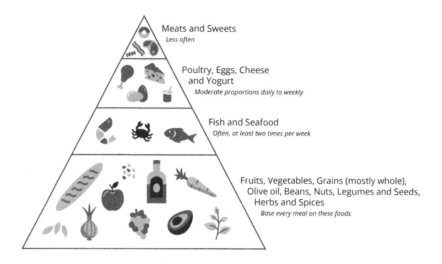

Meats and Sweets
Less often

Poultry, Eggs, Cheese
and Yogurt
Moderate proportions daily to weekly

Fish and Seafood
Often, at least two times per week

Fruits, Vegetables, Grains (mostly whole),
Olive oil, Beans, Nuts, Legumes and Seeds,
Herbs and Spices
Base every meal on these foods

There are some specifics that should be noted.

Cover your plate with two thirds vegetables and only one third with meat or fish. Make the veggies a major part of the meal. Fix them simply, such as steaming, stir frying or baking. Fresh vegetables need little seasoning, although some herbs are both flavorful and healthy additions. Dark greens should be a frequent part of the meal—spinach, kale, collards, arugula, and Swiss chard are good examples. Spinach makes for a wonderful salad; toss it with olive oil and balsamic vinegar and top it with slivers of carrot, cucumber slices and cherry tomatoes.

Fruits are important. Eat a wide variety of types and colors, preferably local and fresh, although frozen fruits are fine. Avoid canned fruits as they invariably have added sugar. Berries such as strawberries, blueberries, blackberries, raspberries and cherries are high in polyphenols that are valuable for many metabolic processes and especially good for the brain.

Whole grains mean just that—not the refined white flour found in most breads, packaged foods such as most cereals, pasta, cakes, pies, cookies, and yes, even pizza. Refined white flour has essentially no nutritional value, so it is essential to avoid all of these, with perhaps a rare treat or two. It follows that trips to the fast food outlet are verboten. Fats are fine in moderation and even essential. Get them from olive oil, avocados, nuts and seeds and fin fish. Avoid trans fats often found in peanut butters (except those made with 100 percent peanuts), margarine and many commercially-baked goods. It is critical to avoid sugar. This is difficult since it is added to so many packaged foods, sodas, yogurts and, of course, ice cream. The limit per day is 25 grams for women and 37 grams for men. To put this in perspective, a can of soda has the full dietary allotment of sugar for a man and is well over that for a woman. One more reason to avoid fast foods. When you buy cheese, avoid ones with food colors; real cheese has natural color. Yogurt is very healthy, but most brands add fruit, flavoring and sugar. Look for yogurt cultures that are "live."

Fish are high in omega 3 fatty acids—the good fats. You need them and can't create them in your body, so it must come from your food. Most beef comes from animals that have been placed in small pens for months and fed a diet of grains such as corn and soybeans to fatten them. This fat is mostly omega 6 fatty acids and is harmful. Unfortunately, the USDA labels the fattest beef as "prime." Beef from cattle that have been grazed their entire life have minimal omega 6 fatty acids and do have omega 3 fatty acids, but the amount pales in comparison to that found in salmon, mackerel or sardines.

Chickens are usually raised in buildings and never see the light of day before slaughter. They are literally stressed plus often have antibiotics in their feed and may be stimulated with hormones to grow larger. Look instead for poultry from farms that use no additives and let the chickens graze. As with all meats, avoid those that have added liquid "to retain moisture." Get real chicken and real beef, lamb, or pork. Still, it is worth being aware that the choline in meat and eggs is converted by the gut microbiota to trimethylamine N-oxide (TOMA) which accelerates coronary artery disease by increasing the "stickiness" of platelets.

Is there anything that you can eat? Yes, dark chocolate, preferably 85 percent cocoa or more. It is inherently healthy. It is also not only okay, it is healthy to have alcohol in moderation.

Buying organic vegetables and fruits and grass-fed meats are more expensive, for sure. But the health benefits outweigh the costs.

You are eating not just for yourself but also for the bacteria in your intestines – the gut microbiota. The 100 trillion of them need nourishment so they can help maintain your immune system and your intestinal lining cells and produce various nutrients that your cells in various organs use for energy. They require fiber that our intestinal enzymes cannot digest as found in vegetables and fruits and whole grains. Consume inadequate fiber and the "good" bacteria are starved. If you eat sugar, refined white flour or too much alcohol, you feed the "bad" bacteria with detrimental results. It is a common combination in the standard American diet, but it leads to increased intestinal permeability ("leaky gut"), inflammation, passage of toxins into the bloodstream, and the induction of a variety of complex chronic illnesses. So, treat them well. The foods that benefit the gut microbiota especially those with plenty of fiber are called prebiotics. There are also probiotics which are bacteria and yeasts that are known to be healthy and are found in many foods such as live culture yogurts, live culture kefir, non-pasteurized sauerkraut, kimchi, miso and other fermented foods. Have some regularly but check the label; only some brands have live cultures.

What about supplements? As a general rule, a well-balanced, quality diet will deliver the nutrients that you need. Herbs and spices enliven many meals and are themselves often carriers of antioxidants and other nutrients. A multivitamin might be useful; vitamin D is needed by many because of inadequate sun exposure in temperate climates; vitamin B12 is often deficient in older individuals because it is not absorbed as well (there is a simple blood test to measure levels of both vitamins D and B12.) These and other supplements should be considered only with your doctor's advice.

Exercise

"Lack of activity destroys the good condition of every human being, while movement and methodical physical exercise save it and preserve it."—Plato

A more modern statement comes from "Time" magazine: *"... the most effective, potent way that we can improve quality of life and duration of life is exercise. The price is right too."* [31]

When a group of mice whose genetics caused them to age prematurely were divided into two groups – one group that exercised three times per week and one group that was sedentary – the results were striking. At the end of five months, the sedentary mice were shriveled, had less functional hearts, coarse and gray fur, thinned skin and hearing loss. The mice that exercised were healthy, indeed as healthy as normal mice, and despite their genetic predisposition to aging rapidly, they did not. This is another example that genetics need not be destiny.

A good exercise program leads to fewer age-prevalent diseases such as cancer and heart disease, along with a better sense of health, less chronic pain, and longer life.

"Sitting is the new smoking." Sitting for long periods (over one hour) is a major risk factor for various diseases, poor health overall and an earlier death. Chronic sitting increases death rates as much as smoking. Inactivity doubles the risk of general poor health. Simply standing up regularly activates the body systems that control blood sugar, cholesterol, and triglycerides. Exercise improves the cells' ability to respond to insulin; sitting increases the propensity toward insulin resistance. In essence, the human body needs to move in order for its cellular and metabolic processes to work normally. Sitting has the opposite effect.

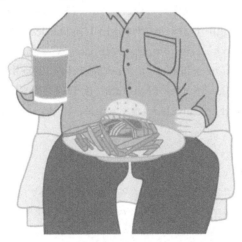

Humans, until very recently in our species' history, moved about all day. It was essential to move in order to secure food, raise children, and protect family from predators. Even in the early part of the last century, most Americans – both men and women – were on the farm, working in a craft shop, or otherwise engaged in daily activity.

It is well known that exercise is valuable to heart health, reduces blood pressure, strengthens and preserves muscle size and strength, reduces blood sugar, and decreases body fat. It also preserves and amplifies brain function and size. In short, *"if it were a drug, exercise would be considered a miracle drug for health preservation."*[32]

Only a small proportion of Americans get the recommended level of exercise per week – 150 minutes of both aerobic and resistance exercise. What is also important is not just to schedule some time each day – although that is clearly advisable – but all day long get up and move about at least every hour for 5-10 minutes. Remember that exercise improves all body functions, not just muscles. For example, it benefits the structure and function of skin, heart, lungs, even eyes—every part of the body.

You already know that exercise has been well documented to help prevent the most important age-prevalent diseases such as heart and lung disease, cancer, dementia, and diabetes. The reduction in prevalence is "dose dependent," as in, the more exercise (up to a point), the less the disease rate. Too much exercise is not healthy, but as a general rule, most individuals will never get to the "too much" level. More than 100 minutes of moderate-intensity exercise per day is probably of no value in reducing age-prevalent disease.

At the other end, is there a lower limit below which exercise is of no particular value? The answer is probably "no," but it is clear that even short bouts of activity are valuable. That said, it is certainly best to obtain the recommended intervals. Less is still valuable, but more is definitely much better.

"Physical activity is one of the best modifiable factors for the prevention of noncommunicable disease and mortality."[33]

Here are the basics that everyone should follow:

- Start with aerobic exercise for 30 minutes five or six days per week. The aerobic exercise can be something as simple as walking at a reasonably brisk pace for 30 minutes. It is okay to talk to a friend while you walk. It's even okay to stop and take a look at something occasionally, but it needs to be steady movement and if for some reason you stop for a while, then the moving time should be at least 10 minutes at a clip. If you have a fitness monitor, try to achieve at least 10,000 steps per day. More would be even better. Don't sit for long; stand up at least every hour, more often if possible. Move about before sitting again. Perhaps you can set up your desk so you can work standing up.

But remember the advantage of some "extra push" every so often, consistent with High Intensity Interval Training (HIIT). These are potent exercises that offer great benefit in a short period. Among other things, HIIT leads to improved muscle growth and strength, as well as the production of growth hormones and myokines, which are anti-inflammatory and reduce insulin resistance. They also increase insulin sensitivity so blood sugar (glucose) can be better utilized within the cells.

- Assume you are using a stationary bike. Set it to a comfortable but difficult level and exercise at a comfortable speed for five minutes to warm up. Then push as hard as you can for 30 seconds. Then return to the slower rate for 90 seconds. Repeat for eight cycles. Initially you may not be able to do but a few cycles, but with time, you can build up and increase the resistance level. During the rapid exercise, your heart rate will increase, and you will find yourself breathing rapidly and deeply. At the end, you will feel tired and will have sweated. Repeat this program twice each week.

- HIIT recruits white muscle fibers in addition to red fibers as in typical aerobic exercise such as walking. Having both types of fibers activated markedly increases the maintenance of muscle mass and strength and boosts your metabolism substantially. It also increases release of growth hormone, which is important for maintaining muscle mass and strength.

- Metabolism is further enhanced during and following HIIT if you are fasting, so early in the morning might be the best time for some individuals. Also, it is important to not eat carbohydrates for about two hours after exercise. Carbs (sugary power drinks, fruit juices, bagels, pastries, donuts, etc.) lead to a rapid rise in insulin. But when insulin rises, growth hormone declines, so it is best to fast for about two hours after exercise to maximize the value of the increase in growth hormone that you worked hard to create.

Add resistance or weight-bearing exercise two to three times per week.

- You may have been told in the past to set the weight at a level that you can do between 8-10 repetitions before tiring. Trying to exert maximal effort for a limited number of repetitions may not be the best approach for some older persons. It may be better to lower the resistance a bit and do more repetitions. But if you can do it safely, set the weight to a level where you can do a max of 8-12 repetitions. As with HIIT, this level of exercise recruits the white muscle fibers in addition to the red fibers and is much more likely to assist with preservation and even increasing muscle mass and strength.

- Although certainly helpful, a gym with weight machines and barbells and dumbbells are not fully necessary. You can use your body weight as the resistance with pushups, sit ups, squats, the plank or by engaging in yoga, Tai Chi or a similar practice. What is most important is that you do it regularly.

- Add in balance exercises two to three times per week. Recall that balance depends upon a combination of brain integration of proprioception (the sense of where your joints are positioned), vestibular (the sense of where your head is that comes from the inner ear semicircular canals), and vision (including depth perception). All three decline with age, but exercises improve them substantially. Try walking a straight line by placing one heel directly in front of the toes of the other foot. This is a good measure of overall balance; you want to be able to walk a straight line some distance without losing your balance. Another balance exercise is to stand 12 inches in front of a wall with your feet about 18 inches apart. Touch your fingers to the wall. Once you are feeling stable and with your weight balanced on the balls and heels of each foot, then close your eyes. Do this for about 30 seconds. If you are comfortable, let your arms drop to your sides and then close your eyes for another 30 seconds. Next, move your feet until they are about four inches apart and repeat these exercises. Next, move your left foot forward and right backward, each about six inches. Get stable on both feet and then repeat the exercises as before. Then reverse the positions of your feet and repeat. With practice, you will find your balance improves nicely.

- Also, it is good to include stretching exercises before and after exercise, and consider participating in a yoga class. These help reduce chronic stress, as does exercise in general.

SLOWING THE PROCESS

"SITTING IS THE NEW SMOKING"

Aerobic 30 min 5 Days / Week
Resistance (Weights) 2-3 / Week
Balance-2-3 Times / Week

If starting an exercise program, it is important to review it with your physician in advance. There may be some approaches mentioned here that the doctor will discourage you from doing based on your health, so do that review now. Start out slowly; there is no need to create sore muscles. Find a setting that feels appropriate for your needs and personality. Although most people find exercise stimulating and relaxing, it may not seem that way at first, so you may need to overcome an emotional barrier. A personal trainer might be valuable, especially at first. He or she can give you good advice, help you devise a program that works for your needs and personality, and "keep you accountable" —in a nonjudgmental manner.

It is worth repeating that sitting is unhealthy. Get up. Move around. "Sitting is the new smoking," so don't let it get you.

Chronic Stress

Stress is a part of life and seems to be intruding more and more.

Chronic stress releases epinephrine (adrenaline), cortisol and multiple other chemicals in a low and steady state—an unnatural condition.

These are chemicals designed to alter body chemistry acutely to respond to an immediate danger such as a truck careening toward you. You cannot fight it, so you must take flight—immediately. We have all felt the rapid heart rate and other symptoms of this fight-or-flight response. With chronic stress, the low but elevated epinephrine levels lead to a rise in heart rate, respiratory rate and blood pressure, which can predispose you to heart attacks, kidney damage, and strokes. Elevated cortisol raises blood glucose, converts fats and carbohydrates to energy, elevates appetite and leads to abdominal weight gain (which is a risk factor for cardiovascular disease). It also depresses the immune system, which leads to more infections and disrupts sleep patterns, which leads to poor concentration, injury, and illness. Asthma attacks can be increased in frequency and severity, and emotions can swing widely with anxiety and depression. Chronic stress adversely affects bone mineral density, predisposing the body to osteoporosis, and it adversely affects cognitive function, which leads to memory impairment and reduced executive control. Essentially, chronic stress speeds up the aging process. In short, the result of chronic stress is clearly detrimental to good health and longevity.

My friend and colleague, Dr. Harry Oken, writes a newsletter for his primary care patients each quarter. In an edited version of one, he discusses anxiety and stress.

> Anxiety, fear and sadness are harmful to our health. These emotions cause all sorts of common and uncommon physical complaints. Negative thoughts disrupt our autonomic nervous system (palpitations, sleep abnormalities, chest pain, shortness of breath and hunger). Negative thoughts can squeeze our adrenal glands, causing changes in our cortisol and catecholamine levels. At the cellular level, it makes our T and B immune cells less functional, and at the molecular level, throws off the balance of our infection and age-fighting cytokines. Our mind becomes our foe instead of our friend. Negative thoughts beget negative emotions, and then we are unable to enjoy the present (a true gift). Our minds can take us to the future with worry, or the past, to beat ourselves up.

You have a powerful mind; you probably are pretty good at making yourself feel bad, but the same neurophysiology can make you feel good. When we are happy, we feel better. When we are anxious, we may be fearful, irritable, and angry. Our emotions make us think a certain way and then our perceptions become our reality. Sometimes this is good and sometimes this is bad. We can lose sight that we control our thoughts, and our thoughts control our emotions. This is particularly true if we are faced with a crisis: health, financial, family or friend issue. Our perception of the problem can get out of control and wreak havoc with our minds, which ultimately affects our physical and mental health. When we really get rolling, the dominoes are hard to stop and before you know it, we feel like we are losing it. The excerpt below is from a book I like, *10% Happier*, by Dan Harris:

> The Buddhists called this prapañca (pronounced pra-PUN-cha), which roughly translates to 'proliferation,' or 'the imperialistic tendency of mind.' That captured it beautifully, I thought: something happens, I worry, and that concern instantaneously colonizes my future.

Since it is impossible to live in a stress-free world, it is critical to find ways to manage those many stresses that come along.

Chronic stress can be reduced with exercise, meditation, relaxation exercises such as the Benson Method, yoga, biofeedback, acupuncture, massage, and Tai Chi to name just a few. None are difficult, but they do require time, something those with stress seem not to have.

A few more ideas are to actively distract yourself with a positive, enjoyable activity. Practice the concept of gratitude by stopping each evening to consider at least one thing from the day that was positive and worthy of gratitude. It might be something as simple as a bird's song. The point is to finish the day on a positive note. Verbalizing (silently) what you are grateful for today can have a significant positive impact on stress levels and help assure a sound sleep. Be sure that you don't let it become a rote repeated item; each day must have had a positive to it—think about it and express it to yourself.

Be aware if you are constantly telling yourself, "I should …" These are basically negative thoughts, and they build on each other.

Laughter is a great way to relieve stress. Watch a comedy on television before bed or any time of the day. Look for ways to convert a negative thought to something positive. What at first seems like a negative thought can often be converted with some attention. Finally, one of the best ways to reduce stress and its consequences is to exercise; it burns up those stress-related chemicals.

Here is more from Dr. Oken:

> You have a powerful mind; you probably are pretty good at making yourself feel bad but the same neurophysiology can make you feel good. Take 5 minutes and play [some quieting music] and think of something pleasant. Notice how everything slows down, think of how fortunate and grateful you are for all that you have. And concentrate on your breathing; breathe through your nose, nice and slow. The music and breathing will allow you to take control of your mind. Experiment with your power. Think of a conflict or concern you have and you probably will get some clarity to it. Perhaps you will realize that your worry just does not matter. Maybe, you need to forgive someone, or even yourself, or maybe you need to just clear your mind. You may discover that your fears are just based on false evidence (F.E.A.R. or false evidence appearing real, as described by Neale Donald Walsch). Whatever it is, just breathe slowly and be in the moment. You may be surprised how you will feel and react.
>
> It takes work to quiet your mind. This is because many of us have unknowingly taught ourselves to be anxious. We have constructed neural pathways that are very fast and take us in lightning speed to panic, sadness and worry. But with concentration and perhaps meditation, or just thinking positive, we can reject those negative emotions. We can build super-fast neural pathways to take us to a calm, tranquil, constructive existence.

Tobacco

A life of no tobacco is critical. Tobacco has a negative impact on many organs, not just bone mineral density and cognitive function. Everyone knows about the elevated risk of lung cancer, but tobacco also has a major impact on the progression of coronary artery disease and many other cancers. In fact, deaths from heart disease are increased much more than deaths from lung cancer. We just hear more about the latter.

Imagine for a moment two groups of people at age 20. One is a smoking group and one is a non-smoking group, and they are followed for the rest of their lives. It turns out that the smokers die on average 11-12 years earlier than the non-smokers, with death being caused by any number of different diseases. That is a decade of life lost! (The graphic, modified from the paper in reference 34, shows the data for women; men are similar except that they lose an added year of life.) If among the smokers a subgroup of them stops smoking at age 40, they won't make up all of the difference, but they will make up a substantial part of that 11-12 years. If a subgroup stops at age 60, they will also make up a portion of those 12 years, not all by any means, but enough years that it will have a significant impact. [34] So, it's never too late to stop.

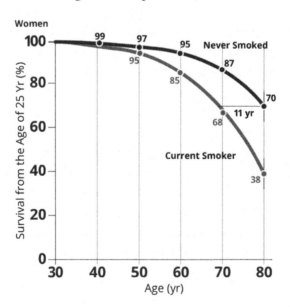

It is difficult to quit, no question about it. Nicotine addiction is exceptionally strong. If you have tried and been unsuccessful, it is worth your time and money to get help from a trained smoking cessation counselor. The adverse implications of smoking are just too great to not give it extensive effort.

Sleep

Part of healthy living includes adequate sleep. About one-third of Americans say they have trouble falling asleep, staying asleep, or waking up too early. Sleep deprivation is common. It raises the risk for hypertension, heart disease, diabetes, obesity and, of course, makes you feel tired and irritable. Sleep is critical for brain health, and persistent lack of sleep can be a predisposing factor to dementia. It's simply not true that older people need less sleep. It is true that older people don't sleep as well or as soundly and may need naps, but a good night's sleep is critical to allowing the brain to flush out toxins. Sleep is restorative.

Older individuals often have difficulty with sleep. There is a reduction in the total amount per night of deep sleep which is important for allowing clearing of toxic products from the brain, allowing memory to stabilize. There is also a fragmentation of sleep meaning that the older person often awakens at night to urinate, sometimes not falling back to sleep promptly. This reduces what is known as sleep efficiency, or the amount of time in bed actually asleep. Significantly reduced sleep efficiency is correlated with increased mortality. Older people also often have a variation in their circadian rhythm such that they become sleepy earlier in the evening and wake earlier than before. This has to either be accepted or possibly adjusted with supplemental melatonin.

Lack of adequate sleep diminishes immune function, along with impacting cognitive function, reaction time, short-term memory and general mood. Inadequate sleep can risk high blood pressure, leads to snacking and hence gaining too much weight, and may lead to drug or alcohol abuse. When we get too little sleep, we tend to crave food, usually the wrong foods. Sleep is critical, yet one-third of Americans get too little.

During sleep, brain cells shrink and the fluids around the cells increase. A pumping action occurs, and the fluids literally wash away toxins and other waste products that the brain cells eliminate. When you wake up, the brain cells expand again, and the washing process largely ceases. Sleep is important to maintain brain cell health.

Here are some clues on how to sleep more soundly:

- Try to maintain a reasonably fixed schedule of going to bed and getting up in the morning. When you go to bed, turn off the lights and go to sleep. In other words, let your subconscious know that bedtime means sleep time—not TV time.
- Have a truly dark room. Turn off all the lights, including your smart phone and any other devices. The light emitted from them, although not all that much, can still impact your circadian rhythms adversely. Keep the temperature no more than 68. Don't be a clock checker.
- It is a good idea to finish your evening meal about three hours before bedtime, so your stomach and intestines have had a good period to process your food.
- Food can help or hinder sleep. Highly-processed foods typically have high concentrations of sugar, along with fat and salt. High carbohydrate foods such as pizza are not good to eat shortly before bedtime—likewise for sugary sodas and alcohol. For many, it helps bring on sleep, but it impacts rapid eye movement (REMS) sleep, which is critical for that sense of "restoration" in the morning. Caffeine, of course, makes getting to sleep harder, so avoid it for at least six hours, preferably more, before bedtime.
- Foods that are high in tryptophan and its metabolites serotonin and melatonin are valuable for sleep and mood. Foods with high concentrations of tryptophan include meat, poultry, milk and cheese; small amounts of grain fed meat, free range poultry and quality cheeses are generally healthy. Serotonin and melatonin are found, among many others, in salmon, poultry, yogurt and some nuts. Rather than worry about which specific foods to eat for which chemicals, it is better to consume a high-quality diet each day. Throughout this

book, I recommend the Mediterranean diet or one of its variants such as MIND or DASH.

- Try to avoid loud, violent or traumatic television shows or similar book readings in the evening; they are the opposite of what you need before bedtime.

- Some quiet music can be helpful, as well as meditation, to quiet your brain. Music with a relatively slow rhythm, about 60 beats per minute, or music that replicates the sounds of nature, such as a bubbling stream or gentle ocean waves, can be quieting. Various forms of aromatherapy can be useful; a sachet of lavender is a well-known approach.

- It is true that something sweet before bed makes you somewhat groggy, but it also gives your body a spike of sugar and then a spike of insulin—not good. Alcohol may make you sleepy also, but it acts like sugar and has a negative impact when its metabolites circulate later in the night.

- Sleeping pills are not a good idea except for short periods of time after a major life stress such as the loss of a loved one. You might want to talk to your physician about using melatonin about an hour before bedtime.

- You can self-massage your hands and face, which will relax not only those muscles but other muscles as well. Certain scents such as lavender are relaxing, so a few sprigs near you pillow or a few drops of oil rubbed on your hands while doing facial self-massage can be relaxing.

- An afternoon nap is also a good idea; it fits with the normal circadian rhythm of an afternoon "lull." Just 10-20 minutes can be refreshing; 30 minutes can leave you groggy. Like your computer, it lets your brain "reboot," or clear out unneeded memories and start afresh. People who take short naps have greater productivity and awareness, less anxiety, and better problem-solving skills. That said, longer naps can help compensate for those who get insufficient sleep at night, though the ideal is to get a good night's sleep and take a short afternoon nap.

STEPHEN C SCHIMPFF, MD, MACP

Other Critical Aspects of Slowing the Aging Process

We have considered a sound diet, adequate exercise, a good night's sleep, reducing chronic stress, and not smoking as critical to good health and long life. That alone may seem like more than enough, but there is still more you need to attend to for quality health and wellness.

Dental Health and Hygiene

As old age progresses, it seems increasingly difficult to maintain healthy teeth, gums and oral cavity overall. Various diseases can affect oral health, and conversely, many oral health conditions can have an adverse impact on systemic or localized chronic illnesses. Poor nutrition impacts the oral and dental health and, of course, dental status may impact eating properly. Missing teeth, poorly fitted dentures and pain may all lead to reduced chewing and the perception that foods no longer taste good. The steady atrophy of the salivary glands ultimately may lead to reduced saliva. This reduced flow of saliva interferes with chewing normally, and accelerates the formation and development of caries (cavities). The mucosa of the mouth changes over time. This can let various bacteria and yeasts penetrate the tissue and cause damage and distant disease in other organ sites. Although the tooth enamel does not replace itself, it does change over time. So, too, do the inner layers of the tooth, leading to damage to the nerve and its associated structures. The gums recede—individuals get "long at the tooth." This gingival recession often leads to greater plaque buildup with its associated microbial populations.

Many seniors today did not have the benefit of fluoridated water when they were kids, so they probably succumbed to multiple cavities as children and teens. Fillings don't last forever, and when replaced, usually must be larger. Teeth with fillings are more prone to additional caries than a pristine tooth. Over time, the tooth may need a crown or a root canal. In both cases, however, the procedure saves the natural tooth rather than having it removed and replaced with a bridge or denture. There is less need today for extractions.

Just like the gut, the oral cavity has a microbiota in symbiosis with the body. They interact and depend on each other. Cavities, periodontitis and gingivitis occur when the microbiota are unbalanced (dysbiosis). The standard American diet ("SAD") that consists of sugars, simple and highly refined grain carbohydrates, and limited amounts of vegetable and fruit fiber clearly alters the oral microbiota just as it does the intestinal microbes. The result is oral dysbiosis. This dysbiosis in turn leads to a state similar to increased intestinal permeability and systemic inflammation. This may be why there is an association between periodontitis and both cardiac disease and rheumatoid arthritis.

All of these changes are a reminder of the need for sound dental hygiene: brushing and flossing after meals, regular (every six months) dental pro-phylaxis (plaque removal) by a dental hygienist, and routine (every six months) dental exams with repair or restoration as indicated. Some dentists recommend an oral rinse with chlorhexidine, Listerine or similar. These are effective against multiple plaque bacteria, but there is a tradeoff in that the overall oral microbiota is altered; it may not be a good idea for everyone.

For some individuals, a battery-operated electric toothbrush can be advantageous along with a high velocity pulsating water stream (e.g., "Water Pic"). Some come with a timer; continuing for two minutes may be most important.

Dry mouth is common and often a side effect of a medication. If the drug(s) can't be replaced, drinking lots of water may be best followed by artificial saliva, chewing gum or lozenges with xylitol.

Vaccines

Certain vaccines are essential for older people. Annually, 140,000-700,000 people go to the hospital with influenza, with 12,000-56,000 deaths in recent years, mostly among the elderly. Influenza spreads from person to person, so anyone who lives in close proximity to others is at risk – especially in a retirement community, nursing home, or assisted living facility – or is in contact with young children who interact with others in school and play groups. The influenza virus changes every year, so an annual vaccination is essential.

Shingles, or herpes zoster, is caused by the same virus that causes chick-enpox. After chickenpox as a youngster, the virus settles in nerve cells and can be reactivated years later when immune function falls—as a result of aging, illness, or immune suppressing therapy. Nearly one-half of adults over age 65 develop shingles during their lifetimes. Shingles is painful and the pain can be persistent for years. The Merck shingles vaccine is effective, preventing about 50 percent of cases and rendering the remainder much milder. A new vaccine from Glaxo appears to be superior to the Merck vaccine. Early data suggests it may protect as many as 98 percent of older individuals. Less clear is how often the shingles vaccine should be repeated since immunity wanes over time.

Pneumococcal infections are common in older individuals and are often serious with pneumonia and bacteremia (spread to the blood stream.) There are two vaccines for older individuals. PCV13 protects against 13 types of pneumococci and PPSV23 protects against 23 types. All those over age 65 should get both, beginning with PCV13 and then PPSV23 a year later to get maximal benefit. There is debate as to whether the vaccine needs to be repeated every five years since immunity wanes over time. Children also benefit from the vaccine, and since older individuals often pick it up from kids, vaccinating children has been shown to reduce the frequency that older adults get infected. Still, those over 65 need to be vaccinated.

Often not thought about, but older individuals need to keep their diphtheria and tetanus shots up-to-date—once every 10 years. Most physicians and health departments include the pertussis vaccine with the other two, the trio called Tdap. Be sure to consult with your physician to be sure your immunizations are up to date. Vaccines are safe and can prevent much unneeded suffering.

Driving

For most of us, being able to drive is a measure of independence. Not being able to drive means isolation, especially in our world of spread-out homes and lack of convenient transportation to stores, restaurants and entertainment. Older drivers are in many ways safer drivers. They drive more slowly, wear seat belts, don't weave in and out of lanes, and don't speed. But aging means longer reaction times, visual and hearing impairments, and some memory loss. These can all adversely impact safe driving:

Driving is a complicated task. It requires people to see and hear clearly; pay close attention to other cars, traffic signs and signals, and pedestrians; and react quickly to events. Drivers must be able to accurately judge distances and speeds and monitor movement on both sides as well in front of them. It's common for people to have declines in visual, thinking, or physical abilities as they get older. As a result, older drivers are more likely than younger ones to have trouble in certain situations, including making left turns, changing lanes, and navigating through intersections.[35]

Add cell phones and car radio dials to these impairments that adversely impact driving – and worst of all – texting. Older individuals tolerate less alcohol. Many diseases render the individual less able to drive, such as stroke, Parkinson's disease, and various traumas. Each person needs to self-evaluate their capacity to drive safely, both for themselves and for those that they might injure.

Living in a retirement community can offer some respite from the loss of driving abilities with shuttles, rides to doctors, and organized outings for shopping, entertainment, and cultural events. This is much better than being isolated at home for long periods with loss of social interaction and intellectual challenges where perhaps less adequate food is available.

Fulfillment

It requires a deliberate effort, but it can be well worth that effort. Humans need to feel fulfilled, so don't let the day-to-day chores (such as bills, laundry, and mowing) fill the day. Specifically, set aside time each day and extra time during the week to do those activities that are truly fulfilling. This will be different for each person, but examples might include a class, travel, a museum trip or rediscovering an old passion that was set aside, such as music, photography, or painting. It is all about thriving and not just existing.

A friend told me about a recent experience at church. The congregation expected to hear a "fire and brimstone" sermon, but the Baptist minister told this story: "When you die, we all know that you will be met at the gates by St. Peter holding a book in his hand. Do you know what is in the book? It is not what you think. It is not about what you have done wrong or right. No, it holds the list of the things you could have done that were fulfilling but did not do."

The following poem by Rose Mulligan says it clearly:

> Dust if you must, but wouldn't it be better
> To paint a picture, or write a letter,
> Bake a cake, or plant a seed;
> Ponder the difference between want and need?
>
> Dust if you must, but there's not much time,
> With rivers to swim, and mountains to climb;
> Music to hear, and books to read;
> Friends to cherish, and life to lead.
>
> Dust if you must, but the world's out there
> With the sun in your eyes, and the wind in your hair;
> A flutter of snow, a shower of rain,
> This day will not come around again.
>
> Dust if you must, but bear in mind,
> Old age will come and it's not kind.
> And when you go (and go you must)
> You, yourself, will make more dust.[36]

Loneliness

Loneliness is hazardous to our health, especially the health of older individuals. The definition is perceived social isolation. Perception is as important in the definition as is the word "isolation." Consider being part of a group that is about to start a ballgame. Two leaders are chosen, and in turn each gets to choose who will be on his or her team. If you get called last, or not at all, you realize that your value to that group, at least as far as ball games are concerned, is low to absent. You can walk away saying you don't really care, but in fact you do, especially if the group of individuals is a group you really want to be part of. You feel lonely because you perceive rejection. As Mother Teresa said, "Loneliness and the feeling of being unwanted is the most terrible poverty."

Those who are socially isolated have more illnesses and a decreased lifespan. Loneliness predisposes to metabolic syndrome and diabetes, and depresses the immune system, accents depression, impacts cognitive skills, and can lead to heart disease, vascular disease, and cancer. As a health risk, loneliness equates to the combined effects of tobacco and diabetes. As a result, loneliness predicts both morbidity and mortality.

Loneliness is common. Estimates suggest that as many as 40 percent of older adults living independently in the community are socially isolated. Some of the predisposing factors are living alone, loss of a spouse, hearing loss, and visual diminishment.

Having multiple social contacts seems to be a good way to prevent loneliness, but it may not. Remember how the group did not choose you for the ball team. They are still there, but you are sitting on the sidelines. Loneliness is more of a subjective experience dependent on various personality factors.

This subjective experience of loneliness is important for well-being. It is different from chronic stress or depression, although any two – or all three – can co-exist.

Although loneliness is subjective, some objective measures of loneliness have been devised such as the UCLA Loneliness Scale, which is based on a questionnaire that examines one's perception of social situations.[37] Observational studies demonstrate that those who score high on loneliness have more infections, more heart disease, and more depression. The social isolation that accompanies loneliness increases the risk of death as much as smoking does and more than inactivity or obesity.

What is happening physiologically? There is a strong mind-body connection with activation of the sympathetic nervous system akin to that seen with chronic stress. Cortisol and epinephrine levels are elevated in the blood stream. Vascular resistance is raised, putting more strain on the heart. Genes that code for inflammation are activated, and genes that normally tamp down inflammation are suppressed. Gene activity is suppressed for proteins that defend against viral infections. There is a decreased ability to "recharge" after a night's sleep or a period of relaxation—neither being restorative anymore.

The centers for "executive control" in the brain are reduced, leading to less resistance to, for example, overeating or overconsuming alcohol.

How can loneliness be countered? The most obvious approach would seem to be creating settings with greater social interaction, but this is likely to be ineffective because loneliness is subjective, not objective. A person with many social contacts can still feel intense loneliness. The better approach, and one that studies are beginning to show has efficacy, is cognitive behavioral therapy (CBT). The concept is to shift the individual's interpretation of social situations toward the positive. You can find guides for self-CBT on the internet.

...

To summarize, there is a steady, slow loss of physiologic function in most of our organs over time. It is possible to slow this annual decline, and with it, the ultimate functional impairments. It is also possible to avoid or delay age-prevalent diseases. But in both cases, it's up to you. It's up to you to adjust your lifestyles. Although it is preferable to begin at a young age, it is never too late to begin a preventive program. You can slow physical decline with exercise, diet and reducing stress. You can avoid many diseases via nutrition, exercise, less stress, and by not smoking. You can slow cognitive decline with these plus intellectual challenges and social engagement.

CHAPTER EIGHT

SLOWING COGNITIVE DECLINE

Loss of mental agility over time is a concern for all aging individuals, and the possibility of developing Alzheimer's disease is perhaps the scariest of all the chronic illnesses. No one wants to finish out life in a state of dementia. For these reasons, we will set aside a full chapter to this, recognizing that there will be a fair amount of repetition since the lifestyle factors that impact aging and most chronic illnesses are the same for brain function.

It is important to remember that some degree of cognitive decline is a normal process of aging, whereas Alzheimer's is a disease. They're closely linked but different. Both can be addressed with lifestyle adjustments, but Alzheimer's disease requires more.

Recall that there is a process in every organ in the body of building up and breaking down. For example, in the bones there are osteoblasts and osteoclasts. Osteoblasts build up the strength of the bone, and the osteoclasts break it down. As children, the osteoblasts dominate and build stronger bones. At about the age of 20, the osteoclast and the osteoblast activity balance out. But then by about the age of 40 or perhaps sooner, the osteoclasts take precedence and bone slowly but surely weakens at a rate of about 1 percent per year. Finally, if the person lives long enough, the odds increase for osteoporosis and the chance of a fracture if one falls.

The brain is no different. There is a normal process of building up and breaking down the synapses (synapses are the connections between the brain cells called neurons, the site where a message is transferred from one cell to the other). This is what allows for brain plasticity, or the ability for new circuits to be created over time. For instance, the brain circuits build rapidly in children, who often have intense curiosity. In young adults, there is a balance, and then, just as with the bones, the decline begins, and more synapses are destroyed than created. Fortunately, the brain, like most organs, has immense reserve or redundancy, but eventually a degree of loss is reached in which there is now a functional impairment. You realize that you are not as sharp as before.

As with every other organ, use it or lose it. The brain responds to challenges and new information with new synapses. Supplying the brain with healthy nutrients and limiting toxins helps this process. It sounds easy, but this can be difficult in a society in which the standard diet is immensely damaging to brain and body, the beneficial chemical releases from exercise are minimal, stress creates toxic compounds and inflammation, lack of sleep limits waste product removal from the brain, and multiple foods damage the gut lining. This leads to chronic inflammation and damage to the blood-brain barrier. Add to this the damage from chronic infections and the impact of toxic chemicals from molds or the effect of heavy metals such as mercury, and it is no wonder that cognitive decline and Alzheimer's are on the rise and rapidly becoming a common cause of disability and death.

Normal Cognitive Decline

The normal cognitive decline of aging can be slowed – but not stopped – with appropriate lifestyle approaches. The "Big Five" discussed for slowing physical decline are equally important to slow cognitive decline. Don't smoke. Reduce stress. Get a good night's sleep. Exercise often and eat a quality diet in moderation. The brain needs these plus cognitive stimuli, including social engagement and intellectual challenge. Here are some examples of how these factors have been studied.

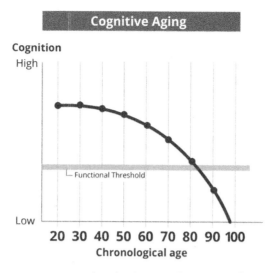

Cognitive Aging

Cognition

High

Low

20 30 40 50 60 70 80 90 100

Chronological age

Functional Threshold

It would appear an approach to having good cognitive function in later life is to choose parents with good genes to pass on to you, along with a nurturing, supporting and educational bent to child raising. In 1932 and 1947, all 11-year-old children in Scotland took a standardized IQ test. Those data have been analyzed in conjunction with IQ and other tests repeated a few years ago among 1,641 surviving, willing participants. IQ level at age 11 was an important factor that predicted cognitive function many years later at ages 78 and 93.

Many of the factors that predispose to heart attacks and strokes are the same ones that predispose to cognitive decline. High blood pressure, obesity, high blood sugar, tobacco use, chronic stress and metabolic syndrome, (defined as any three of high blood pressure, high triglycerides, high blood sugar, central/abdominal obesity and low "good" HDL cholesterol) all predispose to heart attacks, strokes, and dementia. It behooves everyone to deal with these predisposing conditions to prevent these and other important and debilitating diseases. It is known that we should have a sound diet, lots of exercise, reduce stress, moderate alcohol consumption and totally avoid tobacco. If these are not enough to counter high blood pressure, high cholesterol or elevated blood sugar, it is appropriate to obtain prescriptions for blood pressure medications, statins, and diabetes drugs. But remember—lifestyle alterations are more potent than drugs. Pharmaceuticals should be used only if lifestyle modifications are insufficient.

Brain Plasticity

The brain is not just a computer or "hardware" that wears out over time. For decades, it was assumed that the brain circuits are laid down in infancy and childhood and then fixed until death. If damaged with trauma or stroke, then there was little hope of repair. It turns out that the opposite is true. The brain is actually "plastic," meaning that it constantly creates, destroys and recreates brain circuits, i.e. creates and destroys synapses. Each neuron can have as many as 5,000 input synapses and one outgoing synapse. Considering how many neurons are in the brain, this means there is potential for about one quadrillion circuits. A quadrillion is much too great a number for most of us to comprehend, but it is obviously exceptionally large. Usage leads to stimulation, which in turn encourages new synapses to form with new circuits and this continues in the elder years, albeit at a slower rate.

As with muscles, the proper concept is "use it or lose it." It turns out that "use it" is more than mental gymnastics; it includes physical exercise along with the other basics of lifestyle modifications discussed in the last chapter. The brain is not inanimate or fixed but desirous of stimulation. In effect, this is a "message of hope" to all who desire to maintain their cognitive abilities—there is indeed hope to retain intellectual capacities.

Brain Reserve

Brain reserve means basically that one can build up brain function early in life just as one builds up bone or muscle strength. A good education is critical here; education defined in the broadest sense, not necessarily years in school. The brain responds rapidly during early life, so what happens for these first 25 years is critical. If brain reserve is higher at age 20-25, the time when it normally reaches its peak, then it will take longer to reach a functional impairment level as a result of that relentless decline that begins at about age 40 or earlier. Just as it behooves us to build up our bones with exercise and diet in our younger years, it is worthwhile to build up our brain reserve. As with every other organ and function, it is important to start developing brain or cognitive reserve early in life.

There are two aspects to cognitive reserve, passive and active. Passive refers to the actual size of the brain and the total number of nerve cells. Larger brains correlate with less cognitive decline over time. Exercise, for example, can enlarge the hippocampus.

Active reserve is the brain having the capacity to function despite damage. Active reserve can be affected by lifestyles actions. It is built up in early years by challenging educational activities along with appropriate nutrition and exercise. It can be damaged by tobacco and chronic stress. A strong active reserve means less functional loss despite normal cognitive decline over the years. It also means that those with Alzheimer's disease will remain normal for more years before the symptoms begin to appear. What this means is that the brain with a high active reserve can still function despite progressive cognitive decline or the damage of Alzheimer's.

Brain Stimulation

Retirement should not mean discontinuation of intellectual challenges or social engagement. Some form of social interaction on a regular basis is one of the best ways to maintain brain stimulation. In addition to social interaction, individual actions should challenge the brain. It follows that professions with continuing complex requirements are associated with greater cognitive reserves than those whose work requires less intellectual effort and challenge. Some studies have shown that people who attend worship services regularly live longer. Perhaps this is a function of faith – those who are comforted by their faith feel less stress and fear death less. Churches today are vestiges of "villages," so the longer life may also relate to the social interaction of the group that attends services and the social functions that are associated. Other long-term follow-up studies have shown that individuals with more social or interpersonal activity have better cognitive function than those with fewer interactions.

What about so-called brain exercises? This is controversial, but in at least one study, mental challenge exercises (chess, learning a new language, etc.) done regularly showed benefits as long as 10 years later. Brain exercises on computers via the Internet have received challenges recently, and one company was fined $2 million for deceptive advertising. A recent report of one type of computer training, however, is intriguing. It has been built as a sort of game in which the user stares at the center of the screen and concurrently tries to recognize a peripheral object. As the game proceeds, the speed increases. The concept is to improve one's ability to process visual information while expanding the useful field of view (UFOV). In other words, it is designed to help improve the visual area over which one can make quick decisions. Since UFOV declines with age, as with so many other bodily functions, and affects abilities such as driving, there are substantial advantages to slowing the process or even reversing it. The study was called the Advanced Cognitive Training in Vital Elderly, or "ACTIVE," and included 2,832 healthy individuals aged 65-94 at the investigation's start. Individuals were randomized to one of three groups, including one that had 10 one-hour training sessions over five weeks and then booster sessions a year later and three years after for a subgroup. The two control groups did either memory training or reasoning exercises. Overall, the study showed that the speed training reduced the risk of developing dementia over the next 10 years by 38 percent after the 10 sessions and by nearly 50 percent for those who completed the follow-up training, both as compared to the control group. The basic system is available online as "Double Decision," but it is important to note that the study is still preliminary as of this writing.

Creative endeavors are especially useful in preventing decline, whether that's art, music, writing, or other activities. The creative aspect is the most important part, whether you are good at it or not, as well as doing it regularly and frequently.

For the person with some memory loss, music can help recall past memories, so an iPod with individualized appropriate music can do wonders.

Our brains need constant stimulating activities, and learning new skills helps. They challenge the brain and help it build new neural pathways. Remember that once you have learned a new skill, it is no longer challenging, so it is time to learn something new all over again. The important point is to not let your brain become sedentary; keep it active. A book by UCLA professor Gary Small MD, director of the UCLA Longevity Center, may prove helpful to you in maintaining a sharp memory and general cognitive function.[38]

Physical Exercise

We might intuitively agree that mental challenges maintain brain function. But what about physical exercise?

Multiple studies have shown that physical exercise benefits brain function and delays dementia onset. For example, there is a 30-year ongoing study of 2,235 men aged 45-59 from the town of Caerphilly, Wales. Dementia rates declined by 60 percent in those who ate a healthy diet, maintained normal weight (particularly a body mass index of 18-25), limited alcohol intake, did not smoke and walked (or engaged in other active exercises) two or more miles per day. Clearly, lifestyles were critical factors in preventing or delaying cognitive decline.

That 60 percent decline is striking. If the pharmaceutical industry presented a drug that did the same, it would be a true blockbuster. The health implications would be huge, and the profits would warm the hearts and pockets of the company leaders and investors.

Other studies demonstrate, as noted earlier, that regular exercise leads to hippocampus enlargement – that part of the brain involved with memories – and brain tissue in the frontal lobes—that part of the brain involved in executive function, planning and goal setting.

How does physical exercise affect the brain? Exercise produces new neurons in the hippocampus and leads to release of growth factors in the brain overall. Active exercise increases blood flow to the brain, leads to growth of new blood vessels, and protects brain cells.

The amount of exercise needed to drive all of these positives is not much. Before the 20th Century, people achieved it easily by working in the fields, milking the cow and preparing food. Now we are mostly sedentary in the office or at home. For most of us, the World Health Organization (WHO) and the United States Centers for Disease Control and Prevention (CDC) recommendations are appropriate. These include moderate aerobic activity five days per week—though I urge you to try for six days—for a total of 150 minutes, as well as strength or resistance training two or three times per week. Walking is easy, enjoyable, gets you out and about, and does not require a gym membership. yet it improves memory, general well-being and cardiac function. For greater intensity, cycling or swimming improves brain function and cuts depression.

As indicated in the preceding chapter, research indicates that short bursts of extensive effort over time can be effective. Although a nice 30-minute walk works wonders, a shorter time with periods of intense effort, often called High Intensity Interval Training (HIIT), seems to be equally effective (See Chapter 7 for details). "If you are willing and able to push hard, you can get away with surprisingly little exercise."[39] Better yet, if you ride a stationary bike at the gym, do about 5 minutes of warmup and then speed up to your maximum effort every 90 seconds for 30 seconds and then repeat this every 90 seconds for a total of 8 cycles. Do this twice per week. If you push to the max, you will definitely feel it, your heart rate will surge, and you will probably sweat.

There are advantages to joining a gym for resistance training, where there are machines that are safe to use. But there are many exercises that can be done at home using body weight as the resistance. Push-ups, squats, the plank and sit-ups are all good core muscle exercises. Yoga uses body weight as the resistance, and in the process, leads to mindfulness and less stress. Tai Chi, with its slow, steady gentle moves, is actually a good strengthener for core muscles. With regards to gym resistance training, older people cannot lift the same heavy weights as a younger person, and it is not necessary for an elder to try to lift the same heavy weight as 10 or 20 years ago. Find the weight for each machine or dumbbell that you can do for 8-12 repetitions. Don't push so hard that you injure a muscle, but go to your limit. This activates both the red fibers and white fibers in your muscles, both of which need to be stimulated to get the most from exercise and maintain muscle size and strength. Adding balance training to your routine can prevent falls and fractures.

An important question is whether exercise can help reverse cognitive decline once it occurs. A recent Cochrane review of 17 studies of 1,067 individuals with Alzheimer's disease found equivocal results.[40] It was not clear whether exercise can reverse the normal cognitive decline of aging. The Cochrane review did note, however, that exercise keeps normal brains healthy, prevents heart disease, and reduces diabetes and many other diseases.

As will be discussed shortly, it is not useful to study just one element of a program at a time. The brain – like the rest of the body – needs multiple actions (combination of, at least, diet, exercise, stress reduction, good sleep, and no tobacco, along with intellectual stimulation) to maintain its status. One element alone is not enough and likely will not show its value in a stand-alone evaluation. The medical field's focus on studying one intervention at a time has hindered, rather than advanced many opportunities to improve care for complex chronic illnesses and health and wellness management.

Nutrition and Diet

It was noted earlier that central obesity is a risk factor for Alzheimer's disease. Importantly, obese individuals have a threefold increased risk for Alzheimer's disease. An elevated BMI, or more importantly, a high waist-to-hip ratio or waist-to-height is associated with a reduced total brain volume and greater hippocampal shrinkage, both of which result in reduced cognitive function. For instance, the waist should be no more than one half of the height, so a six-foot man should have a waist measurement of less than 36 inches, and a 5'4" woman should have a waist of less than 32 inches.

Among Americans and many other developed countries, the ratio of carbohydrates to fats and protein as calories has increased dramatically over the past 100 years. Especially notable is the intake of added sugars—some 150-170 pounds per year per American. Much of this added sugar is in prepared and packaged foods, drinks, and meals available in fast food restaurants.

The so-called ketogenic diet reduces ingested carbohydrates, including sugar and refined white flour, from the current common level of more than 130 grams per day to about 30 grams per day. To achieve this and maintain the same caloric intake, most people increase their consumption of fats to make up for the lost calories. The term "ketogenic diet" derives from the observation that in the absence of carbohydrates, the body uses fats for energy, converting fat to ketones. Ketones – like glucose – are energy sources for brain cells.

Nutrition is a key component of brain health. Appropriate food is essential for memory, thought, creativity, analysis and focus, as well as various brain processing activities that regulate how neurons interact with each other. The simple answer to the question, "What should I eat?" is to stick with a variety of fresh vegetables, fruits and quality fish in abundance, along with nuts, seeds and legumes (beans[iii] and lentils). This can also include some poultry, a limited amount of meat (grass fed, not corn fed), and almost no simple sugars (table sugar, honey, high fructose corn syrup). In other words, follow the Mediterranean diet or one of its close relatives such as the MIND or DASH diet. These are nutrient dense, reasonably low in calories, and have an anti-inflammatory effect, which is important for the brain as well as the body.

A few specifics repeated from the earlier chapter: Remember that the Mediterranean diet calls for whole grains, not refined white flour as in most baked goods. Healthy fats are important for brain health. Omega 3 fatty acids such as docosahexaenoic acid (DHA) as are found in cold water fin fish are a key component of the cell membranes of neurons. That is why infant formulas have added DHA. Choline is another important nutrient for neuronal activity, and it rids the body of homocysteine, which adds to the risk of both neurological and cardiac disease. A quality diet will contain choline in adequate amounts. Flavonoids, found especially in colorful fruits (e.g., blueberries and apples) and vegetables (e.g., peas, carrots, beets), have an antioxidant capacity that breaks down free radicals that damage brain cells.

What's the proof? Most evaluations have been done in combination with exercise and other interventions, but overall the data suggests that nutrition plays an important role in slowing the onset of cognitive decline.

A Rush University study compared three dietary interventions – the Mediterranean diet, the DASH diet, and the MIND diet – on cognitive function over a period averaging 4.5 years. The 923 participants were aged 58-98. The MIND diet is a variation of the Mediterranean diet with an added emphasis on the polyphenols found in berries such as blueberries and strawberries and green leafy vegetables such as spinach, arugula and kale. The DASH diet is also a modification of the Mediterranean diet adjusted to account for reduced salt intake, along with added nutrients thought to be effective in reducing high blood pressure. Those who followed their

---

[iii] Beans sometimes get a bum rap because they contain lectins and phylates. The key is to soak the beans overnight, replace the water and cook them thoroughly the next day. This removes most of both.

assigned diet most closely had significantly less development of modest cognitive impairment and even Alzheimer's disease onset than those who did not. Among those who most closely followed their diet, the MIND diet was the most effective in reducing the onset of cognitive decline or Alzheimer's disease.

A Finnish study evaluated a combination of a modification of the Mediterranean diet, exercise and cognitive training to determine if it would be better than simple health advice in slowing or preventing cognitive decline. After 24 months, a neuropsychological test battery composite score was 25 percent better in the intervention group.

In a study of individuals 55-80 years old who were randomly assigned to a Mediterranean diet with extra olive oil, a Mediterranean diet with extra mixed nuts, or a regular diet that emphasized reduced dietary fat, there was, not surprisingly, a reduction in cardiovascular events such as heart attacks. On top of that, those who followed the Mediterranean diet did better on the mini mental state examination.

Repeating again for emphasis, within these diets, the critical components appear to be berries, green leafy vegetables, vegetables, nuts, fish, poultry, olive oil and wine (in moderation) whereas the foods to avoid are added sugar, industrially-farmed red meats, vegetable oils and standard white flour. Prepared and processed foods with high sugar, fat, refined flour and salt content must be avoided to benefit from the positive effects of the Mediterranean or MIND diet.

Notice again that fats are an integral part of these diets. Omega 3 fatty acids are found, for example, in cold water fin fish, avocados, and olive oil. Inflammation-causing and generally unhealthy omega 6 fatty acids are found in vegetable oils and in many favorite or comfort foods such as pastries, donuts, pies and cakes. These fatty acids are in abundance in most available red meat, or grain/corn fed livestock. Omega 6 fatty acids, refined white flour and sugars are the mainstay of most fast food restaurants, so avoid them. Remember that the acronym for the standard American diet is SAD.

It is obvious that these foods that are good or bad, respectively, for brain health are exactly the same ones that are relevant for general health and wellness.

STEPHEN C SCHIMPFF, MD, MACP

There are multiple books available on diet and brain health. One such is by Isaacson and Ochner.[41]

Chronic Stress

Chronic stress releases epinephrine (adrenaline), cortisol and multiple other chemicals in a low and persistent state, which is an unnatural condition for the body. These are chemicals designed to alter body chemistry acutely to respond to an immediate danger such as a truck careening toward you. You cannot fight it, so you must take flight—immediately. To repeat from a previous chapter, we have all felt the rapid heart rate, rapid breathing and other symptoms of this fight-or-flight response. With chronic stress, the low but elevated epinephrine levels lead to a subtle rise in heart rate, respiratory rate and blood pressure, which can lead to heart attacks, kidney damage and strokes. Elevated cortisol raises blood glucose, converts fats and carbohydrates to energy, and elevates appetite, which can lead to abdominal weight gain as a risk factor for diabetes and cardiovascular disease. It also depresses the immune system, leads to more infections, disrupts sleep patterns, and causes poor concentration, injury and illness. Asthma attacks can increase in frequency and severity, and emotions can swing widely with anxiety and depression. Chronic stress adversely affects bone mineral density as well, which can lead to osteoporosis. And don't forget—it adversely affects cognitive function, which leads to memory impairment and reduced executive control. If all of this is not enough, chronic stress directly accelerates aging. In short, the result of chronic stress is clearly detrimental to good health and longevity.

There are many ways to reduce and manage chronic stress, including exercise, a sound diet, meditation or a variant such as the Benson Relaxation system or Tai Chi. Don't forget to get a restful night's sleep. Importantly, consider what is causing the chronic stress and then look for possible ways to ameliorate or avoid it. Prevention is always preferable to treatment.

Attitude

A positive attitude is an important precept that delays cognitive decline. Look for successes in daily activities. A positive outlook (recall the Blue

Zones discussion) early in the day leads to increased emotional energy, whereas a negative start leads to anxiety and situational depression for the day. Small "wins" are just as good for your brain as large ones. A simple technique is to smile early and often during the day. Smiling literally helps to retrain the brain toward positivity. Laughing is another positive stimulation for the brain, and it improves the immune system and general sense of well-being. Retired Admiral William McRaven, now chancellor of the University of Texas System, gave a graduation address and then wrote a book, both entitled "Make your Bed." In it, he explains that in Navy Seal training, each trainee made his bed for inspection first thing in the morning. It had to be perfect. His point was that getting something done – and done correctly – just after waking got the day off to a good start.

Sleep

A good night's rest is important, but does poor sleep have a cumulative adverse effect? An increasing number of studies suggest poor sleep correlates with increasing cognitive decline.

One of the important aspects of sleep is "brain cleaning." During sleep, the "glymphatic system," or a liquid cleansing system, literally washes neurotoxins from brain cells. The process requires about 7-8 hours of sleep per day to be fully effective. Among the compounds removed is beta amyloid associated with Alzheimer's disease. In animal studies, sleep deprivation leads to increased beta amyloid concentrations in brain inter-stitial fluid. In a human study, beta amyloid biomarkers indicated that amyloid was not being cleared from the cerebrospinal fluid (CSF) normally during the night when volunteers who generally slept normally were sleep deprived.

Summary: Slowing Cognitive Decline

The keys to maintaining cognitive function and slowing its decline are first to build up the brain's capacity to its maximum early in life and then focus on a combination of a nutritious diet (and not too much of it), regular moderate exercise, less chronic stress, no tobacco, a good night's sleep, positive attitudinal activities and an active and engaged brain.

These are all necessary but perhaps not sufficient; it will be important to determine if other issues are adversely affecting your brain, as will be reviewed below.

A Multifaceted Approach to Alzheimer's Disease

No one knows an Alzheimer's survivor, but everyone knows a cancer survivor.

Medical school and residency training teaches physicians to always look for a single unifying cause to a disease or multiple symptoms. It is often considered good advice. For example, a person with migraine headaches, gastrointestinal disturbances, thyroid dysfunction and anemia may have celiac disease. Alternatively, sometimes a single disease has multiple possible causes or even many causes interacting together to cause the illness.

With more complex chronic diseases affecting greater numbers of individuals and with costs skyrocketing, it is instructive to consider how a multi-faceted approach may be useful for many of these conditions. Often this approach shows that individual actions taken together may be synergistic. It is also important to emphasize that just one intervention may not be sufficient. If the problem is multifactorial – as most chronic illnesses likely are – a multi-pronged approach is mandatory.

Alzheimer's, a neurodegenerative disease, is perhaps the most dreaded disease of aging. Characterized initially by a progressive deterioration of episodic memory, the disease is one of the major causes of disability in later life. About 36 million people live with Alzheimer's disease worldwide—a number that will double every 20 or so years. In the United States, it is among the leading causes of death. About 5 million Americans have Alzheimer's, including one in nine over the age of 65 and one in three over the age of 85. By 2050, this will grow to about 16 million. Currently, it is estimated that Alzheimer's costs about $260 million per year in direct and indirect expenses for care. With no effective therapy, Alzheimer's disease will create even more health care costs and stress on family and caregivers. Of the 325 million Americans living today, about 45 million will develop Alzheimer's during their lifetime if current trends continue.

Alzheimer's is characterized by a progressive deterioration of recent memory. It includes difficulty expressing oneself, various mood disturbances, a loss of executive function (the ability to interact appropriately, pay attention, remember details, multi-task, and manage time), and potential psychiatric symptoms. Although pharmaceutical companies have spent billions of dollars in a quest to find an effective drug, none have worked well. Another failed the day I wrote this chapter, and the company's stock market capitalization crashed 74 percent. No effective treatment slows progression, reverses progression or prevents progression—until now. New clinical trials have demonstrated that early Alzheimer's can be reversed and, by implication, can be prevented. A word of caution. The trials to be discussed here are not the time-tested standardized, randomized controlled trials expected by most peer reviewed medical journals. Rather, they are observational, but the results are compelling. Consider the first studies of penicillin: the results were dramatic, and a comparison was not needed to be convincing.

Alzheimer's disease is thought of as a progressive loss of cognitive function, characterized under the microscope as deposits of beta amyloid, tangles, and tau protein with widespread neuronal damage. But the histologic/pathologic appearance may be only the end product of many different factors acting alone or in combination. As with other chronic diseases, there is often a genetic predisposition. Everyone has a gene called ApoE (an abbreviation for apolipoprotein E, a type of protein that carries lipids), one copy from Mom and one from Dad. It comes in three variants: numbered as 2, 3 and 4. Those who inherit only ApoE 2 or 3 have an approximate 9 percent risk of developing Alzheimer's disease during their lifetimes. The 90 million Americans with one copy of ApoE 4 (i.e., from just one parent; the other being ApoE3 or ApoE2) have about a 30 percent lifetime risk of developing Alzheimer's, and the 9 million with two copies (i.e., one from both Mom and Dad) have a 50 percent or greater lifetime risk. Knowing your ApoE 2, 3 or 4 status in the past would have been of no value and potentially would have caused grief and despondency if you had a double copy of ApoE4 because nothing could prevent Alzheimer's disease.

But now there is hope. Dale Bredesen, MD, professor of neurology at the University of California, Los Angeles, and former president of the Buck Institute of Aging, spent more than 20 years studying Alzheimer's in the laboratory and clinic, and from his own and others' work, he suggested that focusing only on a medication to slow the development of beta amyloid might never be adequate. This has been the pattern of new drug trials to date. He finds that Alzheimer's is caused by a combination of multiple factors that fit into three basic categories: 1) chronic inflammation; 2) a reduction of one or more supportive nutrients, hormones or other compounds important for brain health; and 3) various toxins such as heavy metals and biotoxins. Each of these leads to more synapse destruction than synapse production. In the hippocampus, this means ultimate memory loss, and in the frontal lobes, it means diminished executive function.

In each case, amyloid develops to serve as a protective mechanism. In other words, amyloid is not the cause of Alzheimer's disease; it is a response to various insults that are the real causes. It might even be thought of as a protective mechanism produced to address the insults. However, if the insults are multiple and persistent over decades, the protective response becomes a problem. When the insult is chronic, low-grade and continuous, the amyloid builds up over many years and disease manifests. By way of analogy, think of an annoying cold with a stuffy nose and sore throat. Those two symptoms are the result of the body's defenses—the inflammatory response to destroy the virus causing the infection. Of course, in this example, once the infection is checked, the inflammation dissipates. That doesn't happen with the chronic insults to the brain, so the amyloid response continues. Bredesen hypothesized that understanding the cause(s) and then attacking all of them in a manner individualized for each patient might be effective, especially for those in the earlier stages of the disease. His approach[42] includes not only a basic history and examination but a battery of tests to detect as many insults and imbalances as possible given current knowledge. His team is aware of at least 40 possibilities, and a few more are still being uncovered.

The evaluation consists of determining genetic susceptibility based on ApoE 4 presence or not, plus other known or suspected genetic predispositions. It looks for inflammatory markers such as blood levels of hsCRP (or highly sensitive C reactive protein, which is a non-specific marker of systemic inflammation) and LPS (or lipopolysaccharide levels, which is a byproduct of dying bacteria in the intestines that find access to the bloodstream as a result of "leaky gut"). The evaluation also looks for chronic infections such as Lyme disease, which need to be addressed to stop the inflammation they cause.

As to the trophic supports (some of which also relate to inflammation), evaluation includes elevated homocysteine, or fasting insulin levels, and declines in hormone levels such as thyroid, estrogen and testosterone. It also looks for low levels of vitamins C, D, B6, B12, E, folate, glutathione, and the ratio of omega 6 to omega 3 fatty acids. Each abnormality will be addressed.

In the third category, tests determine high levels of mercury and other heavy metals and various biotoxins such as molds, or mycotoxins. It also includes tests of gut health and the degree of permeability ("leaky gut"), microbiome (intestinal microflora) status, innate immune system status and blood brain barrier status.

A volumetric analysis of the hippocampus is done via an MRI scan as a baseline. (Often this is found to be diminished in early disease but may be regained with treatment.) Various measures of cognitive performance are also included so they can be repeated later as a measure of progress.

Fundamentally, a personalized, individualized approach determines the various causes of disease in a particular individual and then an individualized management plan. It is designed for the individual, not the disease as is so often the case in American medicine today. I am reminded of the words that Sir William Osler, MD, said more than 100 years ago, "The good physician treats the disease; the great physician treats the patient who has the disease." So much of modern day medicine focuses on the disease but largely ignores the patient.

The program has certain basics for all patients. This includes a Mediterranean style diet, including more vegetables, fruits, nuts, seeds, whole grains (no refined white flour as found in bread, pastries, pasta, cookies, cakes, pies and pizza), olive oil, fish, minimal grass-fed meat and no simple carbohydrates, especially sugar in any form. Gluten as found in wheat, rye and barley is eliminated.

Patients are instructed to do 30 minutes of aerobic exercise six days per week and resistance exercise two or three times per week. Reducing and managing stress with yoga or meditation is critical. The protocol, named ReCODE, also includes fasting for 12 hours after the evening meal (as in, no snacks between dinner and breakfast) and waiting about three hours after dinner before bed. An electric toothbrush and water stream ("Water Pic") help maintain dental and oral hygiene. It includes at least eight hours of sleep with the help of melatonin at bedtime.

The remainder of the program is based on the results of the personalized evaluation. If there is evidence of a chronic infection, it would be addressed. If there was evidence of chronic inflammation emanating from the gut, there would be measures to counteract this and heal the gut lining and its microbiota. If there were less than ideal blood levels of various vitamins, minerals and hormones, these would be addressed with supplements such as vitamin D, the antioxidants vitamin C, E and coenzyme Q and vitamin B12 (since many older patients do not absorb B12 adequately) and hormone replacement, each as appropriate for the individual. If toxins such as mercury, biotoxins or mycotoxins are found, then appropriate approaches to rid the body are employed.

Each step in the total protocol has a rationale: to limit inflammation, eliminate toxins, and restore needed nutrients, hormones, and vitamins. The diet aims to be nutrient dense yet calorie neutral, slightly ketogenic, beneficial to gut microbiota and to reducing intestinal permeability. It removes gluten and dairy, which can exacerbate "leaky gut." It severely limits sugar, which is inflammatory, causes obesity and creates insulin resistance. Reducing chronic stress and doing more exercise reduces inflammation. Adding brain derived neurotrophic factor (BDNF) from exercise increases the synapse function of the brain to withstand amyloid disposition. Diet and prescriptions can boost levels of estrogen and testosterone, and diet and supplements can increase vitamin D, folate and B12, which are all important for synapse development and maintenance. Food choices include those with natural antioxidants, but supplements of vitamins C, E and Coenzyme Q may be necessary. Foods with high levels of glutathione help deal with toxins, and specific approaches are initiated to eliminate the sources of toxins.

It is a complex regimen and potentially difficult to follow without assistance. The only real side effect is overall better health. Of course, it does eliminate a plethora of favorite foods and requires attention to exercise, stress, sleep and supplements. It requires time, and that seems to be in short supply for many individuals. As to efficacy, 9 of the 10 initial patients had significant improvement as measured by objective testing, including neuro-psychological tests and repeat hippocampus volumetric imaging that showed significant gains. Among these patients were some who actually went back to work and found they were fully functional again. A recent presentation reviewing more than 100 patients indicated similar results for those with early stages of disease. Unfortunately, those with advanced Alzheimer's disease are much less likely to respond.

Perhaps surprisingly, Bredesen's approach, although initially published in a respected journal[43] in 2014 and presented at seminars, has not become widely followed. Why not? It is well known that new approaches in health care often take many years to become mainstream. This, in part, reflects the time it takes for new approaches to be put into practice widely. But Alzheimer's disease is devastating, and one would assume an effective treatment would be immediately embraced. Perhaps it is just too complex for the average primary care physician or neurologist to consider with limited time to spend with each patient. Perhaps it sounds too much like "alternative medicine." Perhaps it is not accepted because it is not evidence-based on a large randomized prospective clinical trial, or perhaps it just does not comport with the usual approach of trying one drug or intervention at a time, even though standard treatments generally have not been useful. Certainly, it is not an avenue of value to a pharmaceutical firm since there is no patentable drug included. Perhaps most surprising is that the Alzheimer's disease support groups and organizations have not latched onto this approach and pushed for adoption, further studies or widespread trials. Instead, the medical community seems to be saying "interesting perhaps, but more study is needed." Agreed, as Bredesen wrote in his article, but meanwhile no one seems to have taken up the challenge.

I contacted a few well-respected neurologists and asked their opinion of this approach. Each was laudatory of Dr. Bredesen as a highly reputable respected researcher and clinician and they thought his approach was equally laudable but, not surprisingly, each said further studies were needed. One contact told me that Bredesen is "outside" the usual norms in advocating for a combined approach rather than studying one intervention at a time. That, of course, is the time-tested approach to developing evidence in medical care—just change one variable at a time and observe the result. But the downside is that many of today's chronic diseases have multiple inciting influences; unless all or most are addressed, improvement is unlikely. That's been the story with Alzheimer's disease and many other diseases; improving one variable may be necessary but not sufficient. This protocol attempts to address all or at least as many inciting factors as known and as possible. That is its strength.

Before we assume that Alzheimer's disease has been finally cured, it is important to step back and realize that in medicine many supposed break-through remedies have ultimately been proven to be less effective when put into widespread use. The early blush of success fades with time and added evaluations. So, with those caveats, here is my current, but tentative take:

It is a complex protocol and the workup is extensive. Insurance may or may not pay for all of it. But the results for someone with the initial stages of cognitive decline or Alzheimer's disease are so impressive that, if it were me, I would readily spend the money and then follow the program scrupulously. There is no downside except for no pizza or cookies. Besides, the program contains the same advice outlined throughout this book to slow the aging process and delay or prevent the onset of chronic diseases. The key differences are the additional specific steps to take based on the specific insults found to be damaging the brain. Other than the cost of the initial evaluation, the treatment costs are minimal at most.

Perhaps this common thought will now be dispelled: *No one knows an Alzheimer's survivor, but everyone knows a cancer survivor.*

Consider the total costs of Alzheimer's disease today, including the costs of caregivers and the emotional toll it takes on patients and loved ones alike. If this program is continually shown to be as effective as the initial reports indicate, the implications are enormous. Medical costs will plummet, associated costs will do the same, toll on families will dissipate and, most importantly, individuals will retain their capacity to interact and function as productive members of society. Fear can be replaced by joy. It is definitely a message of hope where none existed before.

CHAPTER NINE

A PILL TO DELAY AGING?

Is there or could there be such a pill? Some researchers think so.

According to Dr. James L. Kirkland, director of the Kogod Center on Aging at the Mayo Clinic, "By targeting fundamental aging processes, it may be possible to delay, prevent, alleviate or treat the major age-related chronic disorders as a group instead of one at a time."[44] In other words, rather than attack the causes and treatment of chronic illnesses one by one, it would be better to understand aging, learn how to slow the process, and prevent or delay the onset of various chronic illnesses.[45]

In 1980, Dr. James F. Fries, a Stanford University physician who studied chronic disease and aging, proposed that a "compression of morbidity" would enable most people to remain healthy until a certain age, perhaps 85, then die naturally or after only a brief illness.[46]

Today, the lifespan for a male is about 76 years and for a female is 81 years. Most of us die from a chronic illness such as heart disease, cancer, stroke, diabetes or Alzheimer's. These are diseases that become increasingly frequent during aging and are called "age prevalent diseases." Many of these can be prevented or at least delayed with lifestyle modifications, as discussed repeatedly in this book. Most important are physical exercise, good nutrition, no tobacco, reduced stress, and a good night's sleep. Of course, a pill would be simpler. Too many people are not willing to try lifestyle modifications but would happily take a daily pill.

Some data suggest that medication might have significant impact by slowing the aging process, preventing or delaying the onset of disease or both. Animal studies showed a substance found in red wine, resveratrol, led to longer lives in mice. Other studies have shown promise with a group of drugs such as metformin (a diabetes drug) and rapamycin (used with organ transplants.) Infusing plasma from young mice into old mice has worked too.

For any drug to be considered valuable, it needs to be easy to take, such as a pill. It also needs to be effective, even if not initiated until adulthood, preferably late adulthood. Importantly, it also must have few – if any – significant side effects. That's a tall order, for sure!

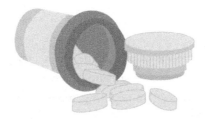

No known drug will stop the aging process, but some slow it down, perhaps considerably. As such, most scientists suggest that anti-aging drugs *might* be able to extend life to about 120 years and do so without the same frequency of the age-prevalent diseases that accompany longevity.

However, drug trials must overcome multiple hurdles. Funding is always essential, but a drug company will not put up its capital unless there is an opportunity for profit, which is not possible with a generic medication. Also, humans age much more slowly than mice. A trial that takes decades to complete is of little interest, so some early biologic mile markers are important to monitor. One such marker might be the epigenetic biologic clock discussed in Chapter 4.

Here are some examples of drugs and other substances being considered.

Vitamins and Supplements

Recall that one of the theories about the cause of aging is that free radicals cause damage over the years. Hence, antioxidants should be valuable. These include vitamins C and E, and coenzyme Q. However, no controlled clinical trials have been developed, nor will they, because the over-the-counter drugs are relatively inexpensive, not patentable, have limited profit opportunities and have high drug trial costs. Second, the most logical approach is to use all three and other vitamins and supplements as well. That would mean if a positive benefit were found, it would not be clear if one, two or all were necessary. You might say, "Who cares" as long as it works and is safe. But modern medicine is largely fixated on determining each drug's individual effect and then seeing if a combination is better or worse. It's a logical but slow process.

N-acetyl-cysteine, or NAC

NAC is an approved compound used in high doses during medical emergencies to detoxify after a poisoning. Apparently, it is safe to use. Glutathione has been found to be critical to prevent age-related stress damage to the cell, but its concentration in the cell declines with age. New research suggests that NAC maintains the cells' level of glutathione during aging and maintains it when the cell is subjected to stress.[47] To date, there have been no human studies, but given recent research, these are likely in the near future.

Resveratrol

In the 1990s Leonard Guarente and two colleagues at MIT found that yeasts with an extra copy of a sirtuin gene lived longer. The presumed mechanism was that resveratrol, a substance found in red wines, stimulated or activated sirtuins. There was initial great enthusiasm about resveratrol. About a decade ago, David Sinclair at Harvard found that resveratrol – when given in high doses to obese mice – led to much longer lives. Almost immediately, a number of companies were established to capitalize on this finding. Venture capital was brought in; magazine and news articles were written. Many supplements containing resveratrol appeared at the local health food store. A company called Sirtris Pharmaceuticals was formed to study resveratrol and similar compounds. Sirtris was purchased in 2008 by Glaxo Smith Kline for $720 million, but then little more was heard or written. Academic studies, however, are slowly discovering the mechanism of resveratrol. Glaxo closed Sirtris in 2013 but continued studies and now plans to begin clinical trials shortly of two sirtuin activating molecules but for just what purpose has not been disclosed.

Wine is a classic part of the Mediterranean diet that includes multiple servings of vegetables, fruits, olive oil, nuts and seeds, which all contain antioxidants. Red wine contains many antioxidants, including the polyphenol, resveratrol. It is found in the skins and seeds that are present in the fermentation stage of wine making but removed when making grape juice. The total amount of resveratrol in wine is relatively small compared to what was used in the mouse experiments, so it is doubtful that red wine alone in moderate amounts or even excessive amounts could have a significant positive antiaging effect.

Sirtuins are enzymes in cells that control a variety of biologic pathways related to the aging process. They do this by affecting the activity of mitochondria, or the energy factories of the cell. Resveratrol is one of many compounds called sirtuin-activating compounds, or STACS, that can modify the activity of sirtuins. This may be the mechanism by which resveratrol has its effect on aging. With knowledge of exactly where resveratrol interacts with sirtuins, it may be possible to produce other molecules that work even more effectively. Glaxo is likely attempting this.[48]

So, the question today remains: Can resveratrol or another similar compound be effectively used to treat humans to a longer, healthier life? We don't know, but that has not prevented the sale of various resveratrol pills and capsules. Presumably, they are safe, but studies are lacking to define the risk-benefit.

NAD

Nicotinamide adenine dinucleotide (NAD) cellular concentrations have been demonstrated to impact both the onset of aging and the onset of age prevalent chronic diseases. NAD cellular concentrations decrease with age but, in some animal models, supplementation protects. NAD is critical for cellular metabolic activities, including activation of sirtuins. Recall that sirtuins are activated by calorie restriction and resveratrol, both known to lengthen lifespan in mice and other animals. The NAD levels' decline with age thus restricts the activity of the sirtuins. It might be assumed that NAD supplements would activate the sirtuins and help maintain some level of youth. The data, however, in animal models is scanty. As to humans, it is not known yet just how NAD or its precursors might be impacted by the intestinal microbiota nor just how it is absorbed and distributed to various organs. To date, human clinical trials have not been done, but NAD is a compound that is known to be safe and can be sold over-the-counter as a supplement, provided no health-related claims are made by the manufacturer. It is available in some supplements today. As with other over-the-counter supplements, clinical trials will probably never be done because there is little profit opportunity for non-patentable drugs.

Metformin

Metformin has been on the market for more than 50 years as a drug to treat diabetes. It is well known to have relatively few side effects.

Investigators in Belgium tested metformin in the worm, *C. elegans,* which is often used for aging studies. The worms remained healthy and aged more slowly. Later studies in mice showed that they lived nearly 40 percent longer than normal. Other research has produced similar results.

Given that, it was interesting that a review of a United Kingdom Registry of 180,000 people showed that individuals with type 2 diabetes mellitus who took metformin lived longer than those treated with one of the other diabetes drugs, a sulfonylurea. Of course, some differences between the two groups may have led their doctors to prescribe one drug versus another. Still, the difference was unexpected and intriguing. It was also interesting that the older diabetic patients (ages 70-75) on metformin also lived longer than older non-diabetic individuals. The groups might not have been similar, but on the surface at least, you might expect those with diabetes to die sooner, not later, than those without diabetes mellitus.

Metformin has been studied in individuals with a high risk of developing diabetes to determine if it would prevent or delay the onset of the disease. In a 15-year study of 3,000 adults, metformin and lifestyle modifications were effective in preventing diabetes. The data is being evaluated to see if metformin also delayed the onset of age-prevalent diseases such as heart disease and cancer. According to Nir Barzilai, MD, director of the Institute for Aging Research at Albert Einstein College of Medicine, diabetics on metformin have about 30 percent lower risk of cardiovascular disease, an equal drop in cancer rates, and a lower rate of dementia and Alzheimer's disease.

Why should metformin be effective? No one really knows for sure, but apparently it reduces toxic compounds released from aging or senescent cells. These normal cells have stopped dividing but are not totally inactive. They put out chemicals that in turn damage nearby cells. Metformin also increases a key enzyme – ATP kinase – that declines with age, and the drug decreases a protein called mTOR, both of which seem to affect aging. Metformin also increases the amount of oxygen that enters a cell. In addition, studies of the gut microbiota of diabetics have revealed a decrease in butyrate-producing bacteria compared to normal. Butyrate is a fermentation product of fiber in the colon that has beneficial effects on the gut lining and immune function and is an energy source for other organs. Diabetic patients on metformin have this deficiency restored.[49] In short, there are multiple possibilities why metformin affects aging, but the exact reason remains elusive.

An FDA-approved controlled clinical trial will test whether metformin, compared to a placebo, lengthens life, as well as whether slowing the aging process will delay or prevent age-prevalent disease. Called "Targeting Aging with Metformin," or TAME, the trial is recruiting 3,000 participants between ages 70 and 80. Various scientists say metformin treatment, if the trial is positive, would become one of the most important therapeutic advances in decades.

Time will tell whether metformin actually has a beneficial effect and, if so, whether it is an effect that is clinically significant. Further, it should determine if slowing the aging process – if that actually happens – will also slow the onset of chronic illnesses. That may not be the case since these are diseases that largely develop as a result of lifestyle choices over many years, but even a modest increase in "health span" would have a positive impact on healthcare costs derived from an inexpensive drug.

Rapamycin

Another drug, rapamycin, also increases lifespan in mice and rats. Rapamycin has been used to prevent rejection in human transplant recipients for the past two decades. Among a series of drugs tested in animals, including metformin and aspirin, rapamycin had the greatest activity in lengthening life. Given the various side effects, however, there was reluctance to choose it as the first drug to be tested in a large randomized trial of drug versus placebo. Instead, metformin was chosen because of its long history of minimal side effects. All of the biologic mechanisms of rapamycin are unclear, but it is known that it prevents transplant rejection by suppressing immune function. Among the anti-aging mechanisms being evaluated are its ability to eliminate adverse cellular byproducts, improve energy metabolism via the mitochondria, reduce inflammation and augment stem cell activity.

Since there is appropriate anxiety about using rapamycin in humans without more data on its antiaging effects, some clinical trials are underway with companion dogs. Dogs develop many of the same age-prevalent diseases as humans but over a much shorter lifetime. Hence, rapamycin is being evaluated for its effect on lifespan, cardiac function, cancer onset and immune function.

Myostatin Inhibiting Drugs

Myostatin is a protein that limits muscle size by inhibiting the size and number of muscle fibers. Researchers at Johns Hopkins knocked out (as in disabled) the gene for myostatin in mice and found the mice developed abnormally large skeletal muscles – like body builder mice. A few drug companies have produced monoclonal antibodies to inhibit myostatin with the intent of treating muscular dystrophies. To date, these have had relatively low efficacy. Now they are being tested to overcome the sarcopenia of old age. In one study, "older weak fallers," or men older than 75 who had recently fallen, were treated with an anti-myostatin antibody. Muscle size increased, which is potentially valuable in preventing bone fracture should they fall again. But like resveratrol, the anti-myostatin drugs were heralded with much fanfare at first but have had limited efficacy so far.[50]

Blood, Plasma and Blood-borne Compounds

Platelet Rich Plasma (PRP) is blood plasma with concentrated platelets, which prevent bleeding. It is used to treat patients with low platelet counts, such as leukemia patients who have aggressive treatment. It helps them clot blood until their bone marrow can make platelets again. It can also accelerate the healing of damaged blood vessels and bone. The assumption is that the plasma contains hormones or cytokines that trigger growth and maturation of various tissues including bones, muscles and blood vessels. Recently, obstetricians injected PRP directly into the ovaries of women who entered early menopause and no longer had menstrual periods. Some of the women began to have regular cycles again, including one woman who had not had a period in more than five years. The investigators were able to collect what appeared to be viable eggs and fertilize them with sperm, leading to the hope that at least some of these women could become pregnant. Has this approach pushed back the biologic clock of the ovaries? Will it persist for any length of time? Will these women now produce the normal female hormones like estrogen that are greatly diminished in post-menopausal women? If so, will they appear and feel younger? Will they live longer? Or will restoration of increased hormonal levels be accompanied by long-term sequela such as cancers?

Blood and Plasma Infusions

Several recent studies by Dr. Tony Wyss-Coray of Stanford University have infused the blood of a young mouse into an old mouse, which led to cognitive improvement. The old mice developed more new nerve cells than when old mice were infused with plasma from old mice. Interestingly, when the test was reversed, and old mouse plasma was given to young mice, the young mice produced fewer new nerve cells.

In a technique called parabiosis, a young mouse is sewn to an old mouse and the circulatory systems are conjoined so the blood of each flows through the other. After a period, the older mice seem younger and healthier, their brain hippocampi enlarge, they produce greater amounts of normal compounds from the hippocampal cells, and they're better able to connect one cell to another, which is important for memory.

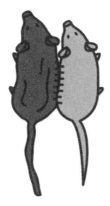

These studies have led to the idea that the blood of the young could have a beneficial effect on aging. However, no one has any idea what the mechanism might be, and more importantly, there is no data to suggest a benefit in humans. It is important to remember that the results of experiments in mice or other animals do not necessarily translate to humans. That said, a number of companies are studying the concept in humans now. Some, such as Alkahest, Inc., where Wyss-Coray is a board member, are seriously evaluating what compound(s) in blood or plasma might have a positive effect. They note that plasma has multiple proteins that change with aging, which suggests a possible link to follow.

Human studies are also beginning. For example, Ambrosia, Inc., a Silicon Valley company, is recruiting young blood donors to supply material to infuse into individuals over age 35. They charge $8,000 for the participant and plan on 600 enrollees. That will gross $4.8 million to conduct the study, which will, among other things, measure biomarkers of aging. This is an unusual approach to science, asking research participants to "pay to play," especially when the investigation is billed not as an efficacy study but a Phase I safety study.[51] Phase I refers to the first human trials of a new drug, where the principal purpose is to determine safety by beginning with low and then escalating dosages.

The Ambrosia study has raised ethical concerns by many, including Wyss-Coray. But the company founder and lead investigator, Jesse Karmazin, M.D., rebuts by saying that plasma is readily available and approved by the FDA (although not for this purpose). He also argues that substantial data shows young people's plasma has an effect on aging and that the only way for him to do the study is to charge. When asked why there is not a placebo control, he said individuals would not pay to be in the control group, and in any event, they are their own controls given that physiologic parameters and biomarkers will be studied pre- and post-infusion.[52]

Alkahest is conducting its own human study in conjunction with Stanford University. The plan is to infuse plasma from young volunteers into 18 patients with Alzheimer's disease. This is also a Phase 1 study; the plan is to monitor cognitive function in addition to safety data. Patients do not pay to participate.

A study in South Korea at Bundang CHA Hospital is evaluating, in a Phase 1 study, whether umbilical cord blood stem cells and plasma infused into individuals over age 55 can prevent or ameliorate frailty through boosting immune function and muscle strength.

Pharmacologic Preservation of Telomere Length with Male Hormone Therapy

Telomeres are repeating nucleotide sequences at the ends of the chromosomal DNA. They naturally get shorter with each cell division, and when they get down to a certain length, the cell can no longer divide and either becomes senescent or dies. Telomerase is an enzyme that helps to lengthen the telomeres. It is expressed in cells in the embryo and fetus but in only reduced concentrations in most cells after birth.

Stem cells, such as blood forming cells and other rapidly dividing tissues, still have modest levels of telomerase, but in the disease aplastic anemia, the telomerase levels in the stem cells are markedly decreased. Aplastic anemia, the result of gene mutations, means the telomeres shorten faster than expected, leading to bone marrow depletion.

Certain hormones increase telomerase activity. In a recent study, the steroid danazol—a synthetic male hormone—was tested for a period of two years among patients with aplastic anemia with reduced telomerase. Normally, an adult stem cell should have about 7,000-9,000 base pairs for each telomere. These are normally lost at a rate of about 50-60 each year, but those with mutations may lose much more, perhaps 100-300 base pairs per year. This is because the telomerase activity is too low to slow the rate of loss. With increased telomerase secondary to the danazol, the patients gained an average (with wide variation) of 386 base pairs during the two-year study. This normalization—and even reversal—of the leukocyte telomere attrition rate was associated with an improvement in the aplastic anemia and increases of hemoglobin concentration, leukocyte count and platelet count.[53]

The danazol was effective for these disease-burdened individuals, but it is not clear whether normal individuals would want to take this or similar drugs since they have significant other effects, not all advantageous. But it is proof of a principle that telomerase activity can be stimulated with biologically active drugs and result in a beneficial response.

This study does not suggest that men should get supplemental shots of testosterone to delay aging and its effects. A series of seven studies called the Testosterone Trials (TTrials) evaluated the effects of a 12-month course of testosterone gel patches on cognitive function, anemia, bone density, cardiovascular status, sexual function, vitality and physical function. Participants had low levels of testosterone for their age but not due to disease, which mirrored patients who are routinely given testosterone today despite zero clinical trial evidence of efficacy or long-term safety. These studies attempt to determine whether testosterone is being administered appropriately. The results so far say there may be a modest increase in sexual function and some increase in hemoglobin for those with anemia, but there is no improvement in physical function or cognitive function. Cardiovascular evaluation was problematic and concerning. Participants had CT scans of their coronary arteries at the beginning and end of the 12 months. The CT scan was able to measure the degree of plaque in the arteries, or the degree of atherosclerosis. Total plaque and noncalcified plaque were substantially increased in the testosterone-treated individuals as compared to those taking the placebo. Calcified plaque, which is of greater concern, did not increase. Still, the findings are concerning. One reviewer noted, "... an unprecedented drug effect and appears ominous in signifying accelerated atherosclerosis." He also pointed out that age-related low testosterone is often due to obesity and would thus be better addressed with lifestyle interventions.[54]

...

Drug companies, up to now, have not put much interest into anti-aging drugs for three reasons. First, the knowledge base upon which to develop such drugs has not been available. Second, natural compounds such as anti-oxidants and generic drugs such as metformin don't offer much opportunity for profit. Third, it has been unclear if the FDA would approve an indication labeled "anti-aging." But this is rapidly changing. The knowledge base is growing, patentable drugs look increasingly promising, and the FDA has now given the green light for the metformin trial.

Still, much is unknown, and it's especially important to learn if there is actually a "longevity dividend," or fewer chronic diseases in addition to longer life.

The business opportunities are obviously great. Conceptually, firms see that if anti-aging compounds also prevent age-prevalent diseases, then they can sell them effectively as drugs to reduce total health care expenses. Given the profit motive of capitalism, the pressure for high prices will be great. But with such a large potential market worldwide, the possibility for reasonable price points is at least possible.

Before we get too excited about a "pill to delay aging," let us remember that good nutrition, plenty of exercise, no tobacco, sound sleep and reduced stress can and do have a measurable impact. Of course, it takes commitment, time and persistence, but it does work and is certainly worth the effort expended.

CHAPTER TEN

DEFYING AGING

"It is a common belief that aging is inevitable and universal. Nothing could be further from the truth"—Josh Mitteldorf and Dorian Sagan[55]

Some people totally deny that they are aging. Others recognize it but are unwilling to change their lifestyles to slow the process. Others still, probably readers of this book, might like to deny it but are aware of reality and pay attention to lifestyle issues in hopes that they will lengthen their days and make them more healthy and comfortable. Then there are those – and not such a small number, as one might expect – who do not deny, avoid or simply accept, but instead actively defy aging. They do not accept "swing low sweet chariot coming for to carry me home." They want none of that. They want immortality. Just like Gilgamesh.

Searching for eternal life on earth is nothing new. It has been a quest of many going back as far as written records survive. In the Sumerian epic of Gilgamesh, the highly regarded king of Uruk seeks everlasting life after many daunting adventures such as killing the Bull of Heaven and overthrowing Humbaba in the cedar forest. He travels to find Utapishtim "for men say he has entered the assembly of the gods and has found everlasting life." After a perilous journey, he crosses the ocean of death, finds Utapishtim and asks for the key to everlasting life. Initially unwilling to divulge the secret, Utapishtim finally tells Gilgamesh, "There is a plant that grows under the water ... If you succeed in taking it, then your hands will hold that which restores lost youth."

Gilgamesh finds it, sets it aside, goes into the waters to take a bath and while there, a serpent rises out of the water and snatches the plant away. Gilgamesh must remain mortal and die. The god Enlil tells him, "You were given the kingship, such was your destiny; everlasting life was not your destiny. Do not be sad at heart, do not be grieved or oppressed."

Chapter 3 in this book reviewed some of the theories on why we age. Other chapters discussed how appropriate lifestyle changes can slow the aging process and delay or prevent age-prevalent chronic illnesses. With such an approach, it should be possible to extend life and health—but only to a limit which seems to be about 120 years. That number is based on the observation that the longest anyone has lived, other than in the Bible, is 122 years. Jeanne Calment of France lived to age 122. She was born in 1875 and died in 1997, having lived to witness truly remarkable advances in medicine and human activities. As of this writing in 2017, the oldest person alive is thought to be Israel Kristal at age 117. Kristal, a Polish-born Jew, survived two world wars, Auschwitz and the extermination of his wife and two children. He then immigrated to Israel, remarried, fathered multiple children, became a candy maker and is said to be thriving today having just celebrated his long delayed/denied Bar Mitzvah.

But can we extend life beyond that? Science would generally say "no." There is a natural aging process, and although it can be slowed, it cannot be stopped or reversed. However, a growing number – indeed, a large number – of individuals believe quite the contrary. They are actively pursuing avenues to slow and reverse the aging process with the concept that humans could live for centuries, if not forever. The Fountain of Youth is at hand, according to some of them. Others are less sanguine but still enthusiastic that the combination of today's science and technology can yield the answers and the actions to take.

One committed person is Peter Thiel, founder of PayPal, an early investor in Facebook, and advisor to President Donald Trump. He uses his fortune through his not-for-profit Breakout Labs as venture capital to seed multiple individuals and companies to do transformative, innovative research. "I worry the FDA is too restrictive. Pharmaceutical companies are way too bureaucratic. A tiny fraction of a fraction of a fraction of NIH [National Institutes of Health] spending goes to genuine anti-aging research. ... [I am] more focused on substance and less on the grant-writing process. That's the direction we should go. I worry that right now, we have people who are very nimble in the art of writing grants who have squeezed out the more creative ... I don't think the answer will be a single pill. I think there will be a series of regenerative technologies and a series of cures for various diseases. I think it's probably a combination of those two that will be the most critical."[56]

Although there are now multiple interesting approaches being taken to understand, slow and perhaps reverse aging in humans, the most advanced are in telomere reconstitution.

Telomere Reconstitution via Epigenetic Manipulation

Laboratory mice have had their epigenetic markers changed and seen their telomeres dramatically lengthened. The process involves creating a form of stem cell that has the elongated telomere without the need to modify the telomerase gene. These mouse cells were tested at various time periods, and it was found that their telomeres began at an increased length and shortened at a normal rate, which meant the telomeres were longer than usual throughout life. Also, there was less accumulated DNA damage and fewer cancers, and the mice lived longer. The scientists were especially excited that the telomeres could be lengthened without the need for any form of gene therapy.

Telomere Reconstitution via Gene Therapy

It might be possible to prevent any number of illnesses with telomere lengthening. The principle is basically to take the gene for telomerase (or the RNA code for it) and insert it into the cells of interest using a virus to carry it there. For example, there are studies ongoing to roll back the damage to the brain of Alzheimer's disease by using a virus to carry the gene to the microglial cells of the brain, the concept being that it is the microglia cells that rid the brain of the amyloid as it is first formed. But they lose their ability as their telomerase concentrations decline.

It might also be possible, at least in theory, to actually reverse aging.

Elizabeth Parrish, CEO of BioViva, observes that a few hundred years ago, we didn't die from aging because we died from infections before we had a chance to age. She is convinced that the technology to dramatically slow the aging process is available and has set out to prove it, beginning with herself as the experimental subject. She says that living longer is not just for our own personal agenda. She notes that we currently have an economic crisis in the sense that older people have chronic illnesses that consume a vast amount of the GDP. The agenda, therefore, is not just to live longer but to live healthier.

More people are living longer—up to and even past 100 years. But for many, those last years of life contain sickness and poor health. Said differently by Parrish, "We want to improve health, and life extension is a side effect of keeping people healthy." This requires finding a way to prevent cells from aging. To do so, she has teamed up with William Andrews, Ph.D., who is president and CEO of Sierra Sciences and a long-time investigator of telomeres. He analogizes the telomere to a shoelace. The shoelace is the long strand of DNA in the chromosome of the cell. The caps at the end of the lace are the telomeres. The telomere is made up of the same material as the DNA, but it seems to have a different function. Telomeres, like the rest of the DNA, are made up of base pairs of nucleosides—adenine, cytosine, thymidine and guanine, or ATCG, the genetic alphabet. When we were conceived, that first cell had about 15,000 base pairs in its telomeres. By the time we are born and after many cell divisions, the telomeres have declined to about 10,000 base pairs. As we age and the cells divide further, more base pairs are lost. When we get to about 5,000, the cell can no long divide and multiply and instead enters a senescent stage or dies.

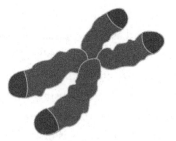

Why does the telomere shorten? Because there are processes in the cell that degrade the telomere's DNA. But there is also an enzyme that restores – or lengthens – the telomere called telomerase. Telomerase is abundant in fetal cells and newborns cells, but shortly the amount decreases markedly and continues to fall over the course of life. What if there was a method to increase the amount of telomerase in the cell? For Parrish and Andrews, that method today is with gene therapy. The DNA gene that directs the manufacture of telomerase is placed in a virus called a vector. The virus is injected into the person or mixed with cells withdrawn from the body and invades the cells, leaving behind its DNA gene for telomerase. The cells now produce increasing amounts of telomerase and, so the theory goes, the telomeres will be not only stabilized, but actually lengthened.

Andrews points to Ron DePinho, M.D., formerly of Dana Farber Cancer Center and Harvard Medical School and then president of M.D. Anderson Cancer Center in Houston, Texas, for verification. DePinho uses gene therapy to take old mice and revert them to young mice. DePinho also has established that most tumor cells contain increased telomerase, which helps them persist and spread.

Parrish is said to be the first human to be treated with gene therapy of this type in an attempt to lengthen her telomeres. Parrish claims some level of success, "reversed 20 years of normal telomere shortening," with no side effects. She gives out few specifics, but apparently the process worked something like this: Her T-lymphocyte – a type of white blood cell that is important in immune function – telomere length was measured pre-experiment and found to be 6,710 base pairs on average, a length shorter than expected for someone her then age of 44 years in 2015. She then traveled to another country where her cells were exposed to the telomerase gene's DNA using a virus (adeno associated virus or AAV) as the carrier. AAV has certain characteristics that make it potentially useful for this type of work. Apparently, it does not cause human disease or an intense immune reaction to itself. It can also produce increased gene expression over a prolonged period. The virus infected her cells and six months later her telomere length was 7,330 base pairs—an actual reversal of the shortening process. Does this make her T-lymphocytes function differently? Does it allow them to divide substantially more times than they otherwise would have been able? Does this make her 20 years younger? These questions have not been answered.

Some important questions need to be answered before we can hope this approach actually works. First, details of the experiment have been remarkably minimal. Second, it appears from what she says that her telomere lengths were measured only once before and once afterward. It would be much better to know that multiple measurements before and after showed about the same results. In other words, how reproducible are the measurements?

Concurrently and apparently using the same AAV, she was given a gene to express a myostatin inhibitor to slow the process of muscle degradation with aging, known as sarcopenia. No follow-up data on this aspect of the experiment have been reported. But success here would be of great importance as sarcopenia is common among aging individuals.

Her company, BioViva, is devoted to gene therapy that "treats biological aging as a disease." She and Andrews have formed a new company, BioViva Fuji, which will be dedicated to further developing and testing this gene therapy approach in volunteers who choose to come to their clinic. The clinic will be in Fuji and the treatment will be rather expensive (amount not stated), but if successful, they believe the cost should decline rapidly.[57]

This study raises multiple questions, some factual and some ethical, and many are not answered since the company wants to protect its proprietary technology. How did they determine the DNA gene for telomerase and replicate it for the experiment? Why did they go out of country to do the injection? Was it done without institutional review board oversight or FDA involvement? Why set up the clinic in Fiji? Is it to avoid FDA oversight? From the web site, it appears the telomerase gene was given in a way to reach blood stem cells. Those are now younger, but what about all of the body's other cells? How did they approach muscle cells to insert the gene to quell sarcopenia? Hopefully, there will be a report in the scientific literature that answers these and other questions.

Ethics, Philosophy, and Questions Related to Denying Aging

As with many new ideas and technologies, not everyone agrees that defying aging is appropriate or rational. Some say that we humans have no business interfering with the processes of death other than to prevent or treat illnesses. Others, of course, say we are imbued with intelligence and it is our right and duty to investigate options.

Several questions to consider: If people can live an indefinite period of time, how will that affect retirement age? Who will pay for it? Sooner or later, each person will presumably develop chronic illnesses as they do today. Once this happens, won't the costs of healthcare be the same, just delayed for some years? Will the planet become overpopulated, leading to starvation, violence and anarchy with everyone living longer times, if not forever?

There are also lifestyle questions. Today, a 75-year-old would probably not choose to go back to school for a Ph.D. because the time horizon to use the knowledge gained would be limited. But what if time were not limited? Will individuals have one career for some time period and then choose to get "retooled" at say age 75 and again at 110 for new careers? Will there ever be retirement if people have to work to support themselves indefinitely?

Summary

There is intense interest in dramatically extending lifespans, especially healthy lifespans. Gene therapy approaches to lengthen the chromosomal telomeres may show modest or substantial effect, but the scientific studies are still in very early stages. Watch for more intriguing experiments to come in the near future.

CHAPTER ELEVEN

HONOR YOURSELF

Doris Roberts of the television show "Everybody Loves Raymond" testified before Congress that ageism is the "last bastion of bigotry."

Probably no one would deny that Americans have a strong preference for the young adult. Older people are considered askance. The desired person is the one with youthful energy.

There is a stereotypical bias against the older person based on the generally held belief that age connotes a loss of status and a loss of role in the community. For many people, older individuals are perceived as lacking in full abilities and therefore not suitable for employment—or even equal attention. The conscious or subconscious perceptions about older individuals may include positive attributions such as wisdom, but most are negative. Older people are seen as too old to work, too old to use a computer or iPad, and too old to contribute. Having a strong age bias leads to assumptions that an older person has certain "debilities."

This is compounded today because older individuals are continuing to work, some out of necessity and others to maintain income, a sense of self-worth, and intellectual challenge. Labor force participation rose substantially for those over age 65 in recent years. Boomers, in a 2015 Harris Poll, indicated that they were the "best problem solvers" but millennials thought distinctly otherwise (65 percent versus 5 percent). Companies, of course, are often happy to help long-time older employees out the door, despite their wealth of experience, replacing them with younger individuals who accept lower wages, expect no pension and whose health care costs are often considerably less.

"Ageism" is a relatively new term originally created to parallel sexism and racism.[58] Some would say that ageism is even more difficult to counteract. African-Americans, homosexuals, women, and those with disabilities have all seen the populace and its leadership show acceptance and institute laws to prevent overt discrimination. Not so with the elderly. Prejudice remains high and acceptable whereas other "-isms" are now perceived as no longer acceptable although often present.

Ageism is unique in that older individuals are of all races, ethnicities and both genders. And those that are biased against the elders will become ones themselves in due course. Perhaps it is a defense mechanism: "I don't want to get older so I will be biased toward those who are."

But others just don't think older people are valuable. Silicon Valley may be the epicenter for such beliefs. Consider Mark Zuckerberg's famous comment "Young people are just smarter." And of course there is the perception that elders are "takers" rather than "producers." They get Social Security and have Medicare, both of which are basically generation transfer taxes which the young are now paying to support the elders. An unfair but perhaps understandable attitude. Perhaps the whole issue is death. Old connotes that death is coming. If one can escape becoming older, then one also escapes death. But since that is not realistic, it is easier to hold a strong negative bias toward the older person.

"Senectus morbidus est," ("Old age is a disease") wrote Seneca, the first century Roman philosopher. That attitude is alive and well today as aging is often assumed to be closely related to disease and disability.

A cultural shift occurred at the time of the industrial revolution. Older adults were "pastured" and marginalized because it was assumed that they could not produce in the work marketplace like the younger individuals vying for jobs. The result has been an isolated older population that is neither honored nor appreciated. To some degree, perhaps to a large degree, it is corporate America that has advanced ageism because it wants to sell its many options to look younger, feel younger, and think younger. By "medicalizing" aging, industry looks to sell its wares to an elderly population that desperately wants to not look, act, or feel old.

America, and much of the developed world, has become a "throwaway society." When a car is just a few years old, it is disposed of even though it may have many useful years ahead. Clothing is even more disposable with new styles pushing out the old in the closet. Glass bottles are no longer returned for cleaning and refilling. Many people don't bother with recycling or composting; it is easier to just send it to the landfill.

America, where innovation, youthfulness and boundless energy are honored, takes the same approach with older individuals. Consider the cocktail party. The first question asked is, "What is your job?" —not what did you do in the past or what are your current interests—but what do you *do* now? If you are not actively employed in a "useful" position, the questioner shortly moves on. You are not valuable.

Strong business interests promote the concept of ageism, although never overtly. The cosmetics industry, the fashion industry, the supplement industry, and many medical interests are all largely dependent on older individuals feeling they need to look and feel younger. These companies extoll the older individual to part with their money in a never-ending quest for youth.

And what do older individuals do? They get their Botox, plastic surgery, hair transplants, and extensive makeup—anything to preserve the appearance of a younger person. Is this unwillingness to age, or is it a defense? Do they know full well that the younger in society will discard them, view them as diminished and therefore no longer be of value?

Ageism may be more overt against women who are taught throughout life that they must be attractive and so find themselves in the beauty parlor and at the drug store counter with anti-aging creams and hair dyes. Plastic surgeons are primarily frequented by older women. In movies and television, an older woman is distinctly uncommon.

Debora Spar, the president of Barnard College and a self-described post-feminist, writes that as a young woman she had breast reduction surgery, noting "although there was some medical rationale for the procedure, the overwhelming reason was that I was sick and tired of every man on the planet being unable to look above my neck." Now she has climbed the social and professional ladder, aged some, and begins to wonder "if everyone must avail themselves of cosmetic surgery, Botox, various collagen fillers, etc. in order to maintain their own sense of value in a world that increasingly worships younger looks ... Or is it sufficient to be satisfied with oneself." [59]

The first half of life is an uphill course of growing, learning, maturing and gaining experience. The second half begins the downhill course, and a point in time occurs when one is labelled "older" by society and set aside emotionally and often physically.

Conceptually, each person would like to "live long and die short," meaning a long life of good health and a short period of decline leading to death. Individuals in their sixties and early seventies, to a great extent, don't want to age or be less physically and mentally capable. No one does. But that is what happens. At some point, a person begins to accept the changes and come to terms with them. Each must decide how well he or she will age. You must be the author of your own story.

But society's view of the elderly is "sick and dying." The societal tendency is to define people by their disabilities rather than their abilities, which likely are many. It is hard for a younger adult to look at an older person and remember that wrinkled face was once smooth, that bald head was once covered, and those thin arms and legs were once large and strong. That aging person was once a child who jumped, skipped, and ran.

It is interesting that children are also defined by their inabilities. With both the old and the young, the adult mindset is that the young's purpose is to prepare for adulthood and that the old's purpose has declined past that valued ideal stage.

But older age need not imply deficiency or a diminishment. Alison Gopnik, Ph.D., a professor of psychology at UC Berkeley, wrote, "You still often read psychological theories that describe the young and the old in terms of their deficiencies, as if these stages of life were just preparation for, or decline from, an ideal grown-up human. But new studies suggest that the young and the old may be especially adapted to receive and transmit wisdom. We may have a wider focus and a greater openness to experience when we are young or old than we do in the hurly-burly of feeding, fighting and reproduction that preoccupies us in our middle years ... Human life history is weird. We have a much longer childhood than any other primate, and we developed special adaptations to care for those helpless children—most notably, females who outlive their fertility. These grandmothers also pass on two generations' worth of knowledge; they are crucial to the evolution of learning and culture."

This idea of the wisdom of the aged occurs frequently in the blue zones, where elders are honored and appreciated. As we learned earlier, these cultures live in fundamentally different ways than most Americans. They mostly walk to work, the store, and church. They eat a nutritious diet and not too much of it. Their stress levels seem to be low. Few smoke. Their social engagement is high. Older people are part of the fabric of society and the family. Their advice is sought and appreciated.

The elderly are often spoken of as holding wisdom. There is much to this. Although the parents must physically raise the children, provide them shelter, clothing and food, and see to their general education, the elders impart wisdom, cultural norms and civility to their grandchildren. To a large extent, this has been lost.[60] When honored in those cultures, their advice and wisdom is listened to and appreciated. But in American society and in many other Western cultures today, elders are "set aside," just as is everything else that is not new and shiny. The disposable society tends to not use anything that is the least bit "old," but instead discards it in favor of the newest, most glamorous, most trendy items. The same happens to older individuals.

In the past, the grandparents lived on the farm with the next generations. No longer. Families are more often than not dispersed in various parts of the country or world. The opportunity for grandparents to help with raising the next generation of children is circumscribed today.

In the blue zones (see Chapter 5), families are nuclear, live near one another and interact. The elders are respected and considered an integral part of the extended family. The blue zone elders – like children – are more attuned and more open to the world around them. Children are ready to receive wisdom, and the elders are there to provide it.

Plus, some characteristics of older people are often not recognized. Elders are more likely to sense gratitude, are more willing to forgive, are more calm in the face of conflict and confusion, and are generally less prone to anger. They can use their years of experience and expertise in life to make quality decisions.[61]

Nursing homes have always been places were the disabled are basically warehoused. Most people I know over the years have stated emphatically that they do not ever want to be "sent to one of those places." Why? Because residents are considered no longer valuable members of society, are discarded, and lose their autonomy and dignity. Once Dr. William Thomas became the medical director of a nursing home in upper New York state, he found residents were "dull and dispirited." He decided to change that dramatically. He brought in two dogs, four cats, more than 100 parakeets, and some chickens and rabbits. He set up a garden, added plants to the residents' rooms and common areas and, to bring young life to the facility, added a day care center for his staff's children. The results were nothing short of dramatic. Residents' spirits were buoyed, their sense of autonomy rose, they became more socially engaged with staff and other residents, they relished caring for the animals, and they enjoyed the children. They began to eat better, drug use declined, and deaths were reduced.[62]

Perhaps it is too much to hope or assume that society will change, and ageism will decline. It is, however, incontrovertible that there will be older people. They may have to fend for themselves. Here are some possible ways to do so in preparation for and during the elder years.

This book is not about finances and money during "retirement," but both are obviously critical. Saving and investing, beginning in early adulthood, are essential. No one can or should assume that someone else or the government will pay for their expenses once they retire. This is especially true as the aging population grows, and the working population declines as a percentage. There are fewer workers to support generation transfer tax programs such as Social Security and Medicare. Large companies and governments are discovering that they made promises that cannot be kept regarding pensions and healthcare. Bottom line: Look out for yourself. Don't assume governmental or employer beneficence.

Elders have social and political clout. They vote and are listened to by politicians as a result. Seniors also – as a generalization – have a combination of wisdom and maturity which helps them achieve their social and political expectations. Stay attuned to what seniors want and need, and make your voice heard, especially in the voting booth.

Think of aging as a process, or a continuum like the first decades of life. It follows roughly three stages: transition or transformation in the sixties, distinction in the seventies, and completion in the eighties and beyond. Will aging be a negative or a positive part of your life? The answer depends principally on your choices. [63]

The transition period in the sixties begins when one realizes that "the road ahead is shorter than the road behind." It is a good time to pause and consider what has been accomplished in life rather than look for new mountains to climb. Work life will end soon, and it is time to take stock and appreciate who you are and what you have done. As this book has emphasized repeatedly, pay attention to lifestyle and change it now for the better if you have not done so already. It is also time to recognize and accept your age. Said differently, be proud of who you are and remember that nature usually creates hair color that matches your skin tone nicely.

Appreciate who you are, not who you have been. Decide what is most important in the next years of life and concentrate on them; put the less important aside. Begin to give greater appreciation to nature and nature's handiwork around you. You might begin a journal. "Self-expression decreases stress and focuses attention," which leads to positive outcomes, decreased anxiety, an attentive mind and improved attitude. If you like, your notebook or journal can become a guide for your grandchildren and a living legacy for your children. This is also a time when it is wise to enlarge your circle of friends. In all probability, many of your friends are largely those at work, but once work ends, they will likely peel away as interests diverge. This might seem like a surprise, but it is consistently true. Having a circle of friends is critical to aging well. You need that social engagement, and it will be easier later if you already have already developed and nurtured friendships now.[64]

Since you have become an "elder," you should accept it and bask in its glow. Don't avoid it. Although society focuses on the young and has a deep-seated negative bias, you need not accept it. Assume the role of the elder and act upon it with your children and grandchildren and others. Don't wait for them to invite you into this new role. They probably don't see or don't want to see you as having aged. It is a gradual process physically and mentally, so it is less noticeable day-to-day. In other words, accept the elder role actively rather than wait passively for an invitation.

If you have been in power struggles with family members, this is a good time to find a process to end them. You can accept and forgive, although you can certainly express your views. In addition to that journal, this would be a good time to write a life review letter to family and friends that are important to you. Developed by faculty at Stanford Medical Center, the goal is "to help, empower and support all adults to prepare for their future and take the initiative to talk to their doctors and their friends and family about what matters most to them at life's end."[65]

The letter need not be long but might include a recognition of those that are important to you, a few memories of key events in life, a note to ask forgiveness from those you have injured, offer forgiveness to those who have hurt you, some "thank you's, "I love you's, and some "goodbyes."[66] This is a way to clear up some important issues that you might have difficulty doing verbally, and which are not covered in a will or other legal papers. There is a link in the end notes to a template you can use.

In your seventies, you enter what Gurian in his book, *The Wonder of Aging*, calls the age of distinction. This is a time to be proud of who you are, what you have accomplished, and what you believe. By now, you should know who you are and what you stand for. Your light should not be hidden away. "No one lights a lamp and then puts it under a basket." (Luke11:33) This is your time to give back to your grandchildren, community, and passions. It is a good time to volunteer and participate. Keep your light out in full view.

In Erickson, Narrett, Kung and Davila's book *Old is the New Young*,[67] they offer four "pillars" and 10 "secrets" to aging gracefully. The Pillars are: Physical, Mental, Spiritual and Financial. The first three have been addressed in this book. The financial issues, obviously critical to comfort and satisfaction in the elder years, have not been addressed but can be found elsewhere.

Their "Ten Secrets," all discussed in various ways in prior chapters, includes:

- It Can Be Done: "You can't help getting older, but you can help getting old," George Burns says.
- Think Positively: Positive thinking helps give you the motivation to make necessary adjustments in living.
- Care for Yourself: Pay attention to diet, exercise, stress management, sleep, dental hygiene—and no tobacco.
- Find Your Team: It may be spouse, friends, healthcare team, children, others—they want to help, so let them.
- Know Your Weak Spots: Perhaps you have hypertension, elevated cholesterol, tobacco, diabetes mellitus, poor diet, or a sedentary life.

Once you know and understand those weak spots, it is time to work on them with the help of your loved ones, friends, and healthcare team.

- Stay Curious: Learn new skills such as dance steps or a musical instrument. Don't just listen but engage.
- Sharpen Your Mind: Improve your memory, and do brain exercises regularly.
- Build Resilience: Augment your ability to adjust to change with a positive outlook.
- Seek Help: You don't have to do it alone. Others are ready and willing to help, but it will be up to you to ask.
- Put Your Money Where It Counts: Spend it wisely and invest where it will safely reap rewards in the future.

These are worth rereading, thinking about and putting into practice. They will serve you well.

At any age, several everyday basics can make life better. Begin with a positive mindset. An appropriate view might be "old is the new young"[68] and "you can have a great life as an elder." Said somewhat differently, aging is not the same as becoming ill or disabled. Having gratitude is important, so look for the simple things each day that are positive. It might be a bird with a beautiful song this morning while you were lying in bed, the smile of a grandchild, or the kiss from your beloved. Cherish each one, think of them in the evening, and review them just before falling asleep. That will help assure a better night's sleep and a more positive attitude upon awakening.

Actively look for ways to maintain and further develop intellectual stimulation, social interaction, community involvement and spiritual enhancement. These are important to maintaining cognitive function, avoiding loneliness, and enjoying life to the fullest.

Develop a set of lifestyle habits as described in the preceding chapters at a young age that will maintain the body, mind and spirit. These include good nutrition, regular exercise, reduced stress, no tobacco, good sleep patterns, dental hygiene, sensible approaches to avoid trauma (such as no texting or driving after drinking), age-appropriate vaccines, and actionable health screenings (such as blood pressure or cholesterol). You may have put these off due to the press of work and other commitments, so now is the time to get started. It is never too late.

Society may or may not honor you as an elder, but you can honor yourself with these approaches. This list is not that long, and doing them will help you remain positive, engaged and healthy. It is worth the effort.

CHAPTER TWELVE

21ST CENTURY COMPREHENSIVE PRIMARY CARE

We can slow the aging process and avoid many chronic illnesses with appropriate lifestyle behaviors. That is good, but it is not sufficient. As we age, it's also important to have truly comprehensive primary care.

We tend to think of our primary care physician (PCP) as the one who does the "simple stuff," a doctor who is a mile wide and an inch deep in knowledge and experience. That is a false impression. In fact, the PCP is actually a "chronic disease specialist." That is true by education and experience, provided the PCP is up to date with the 21st century approach to chronic illnesses and has the time to care for his or her patients with these diseases. Unfortunately, this is not always the case. [69]

PCPs are skilled at managing, for example, diabetes with complications, heart failure, chronic lung diseases, hypertension and obesity. They see patients with these illnesses in their practice daily, so their experience level is high. Sure, the organ or disease specialist is needed some of the time but not all that often when an experienced primary care physician is at the helm.

Comprehensive primary care means a close relationship between patient and doctor. It means dealing with the episodic medical problems that occur throughout life. It also means actively managing serious chronic illnesses. It means coordinating that care when specialists are required. It means helping patients maintain wellness by working on chronic illness risk factor detection and reduction. It means preventing acute illnesses through vaccines and other approaches. When it is comprehensive, it can deal with 95 percent of health care needs. Specialists are rarely needed, prescription use goes down, hospitalization rates and ER visits fall substantially, and total costs of care are reduced. Patients are healthier and content when they avoid the need for medical care.

The key requirements of comprehensive primary care include some basics: a well-educated, well-trained, up-to-date PCP who is committed to relationship-based care and uses a proactive team-based approach. A second key ingredient is time—time to listen, think, diagnose, treat and prevent. This can be especially important for older patients with multiple chronic illnesses and prescription medications. It is equally important for patients with vision, hearing, mobility or memory impairments, as well as those with anxieties that drive the underlying medical issue. These all require time. The third require- ment, likewise essential, calls for an understanding of the new paradigm of managing complex chronic illnesses. This is a distinct change from the acute care model of care that has been the basic methodology for more than 100 years.

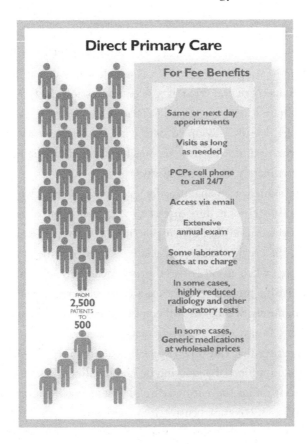

Direct Primary Care

For Fee Benefits

Same or next day appointments

Visits as long as needed

PCPs cell phone to call 24/7

Access via email

Extensive annual exam

Some laboratory tests at no charge

In some cases, highly reduced radiology and other laboratory tests

In some cases, Generic medications at wholesale prices

FROM
2,500
PATIENTS
TO
500

You may have heard there is a primary care crisis in the United States. You may feel it because you only get 8-12 minutes with your PCP, who interrupts you within about 18 seconds and never fully listens to you. Most primary care physicians don't have enough time today, and the result is a tendency to quickly refer to specialists. With added time, however, the PCP could have dealt with the problem. A PCP who deals with mostly geriatric patients should have no more than about 500 patients (compared with the usual 2,500-3,000 of most primary care physicians) and only about 10-12 visits per day (compared to 25-30).

All too often, under today's practice pressures to see too many patients per day, the PCP does not have adequate time to practice as this chronic disease specialist. If there is only 10 minutes for a visit and the situation is the slightest bit complicated, it's off to the specialist. This, of course, drives up cost but does not drive up care quality. It's much better if the PCP sees fewer patients per day – yet retains the same income – and then offers those patients the high level of care that he or she is actually capable of providing. This model has been called direct primary care, retainer-based or concierge care, which are all similar.

Comprehensive primary care offers same or next-day appointments that last as long as necessary and 24/7 access via the PCP's cell phone. Often it means generic medications at wholesale prices and reduced costs on laboratory tests and radiology. It means improved care quality and satisfaction and fewer frustrations for patient and doctor alike.

A small caseload means more time for the patient and doctor to interact. It means more time for listening, building trust, and healing. It means better diagnostics and improved treatment plans. This results in fewer tests, X-rays, prescriptions and referrals. Combined with a much less expensive high-deductible health insurance policy, the savings for patients are substantial and the total cost of all care declines quite dramatically. Putting more resources into primary care is definitely cost effective.

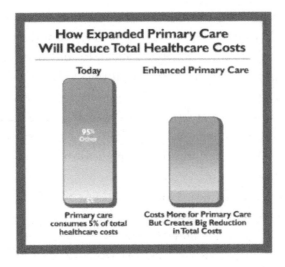

Unfortunately, even if freed of time constraints, not every PCP is able or willing to provide this type of comprehensive primary care. Some spend a bit more time with each patient but don't accept the mantra of "chronic disease specialist." To change health care in a meaningful way, 21st century medicine needs to follow a different path. Some call it functional medicine. Other names abound. The point is to listen carefully to the patient, seek out not just the current symptoms and disease parameters but the antecedents and triggers. These must be discovered and addressed if the chronic illness is to be realistically reversed rather than just tamped down. But today, these factors more often than not are glossed over or just ignored.

Most PCPs have practiced in a certain way for years that has become their standard so becoming a chronic disease specialist with a functional bent is a new approach to practice. It's a new paradigm that they may not be prepared or knowledgeable to follow.

An important question is to ask how physicians can regain time. Simply substituting "value," as is the Medicare and insurers' buzzword, is not the way. It requires insurers to pay more per visit or more per capitated individual, with the understanding that patients receive whatever time is needed. It means that employers should offer to pay the membership or retainer of the direct primary care (a.k.a. membership or concierge) physician or establish a company clinic with PCPs who are not overburdened. It means individuals should seek a PCP who limits his or her practice to about 500-700 total individuals and visits to 10-12 per day instead of 25 or more. You deserve at least 30 minutes for most visits and more for complex issues.

Insurers, including Medicare and Medicaid, are not inclined to pay for direct primary care in the mistaken belief that it only increases costs of primary care. It does, of course, but they need to appreciate that better primary care means lower total costs. Their expenses will go down substantially with a switch to direct primary care models, provided that PCPs follow the general outline described above.

Physicians need to understand and commit to the new paradigm of managing complex chronic illnesses as suggested by the model discussed for Alzheimer's disease. Some will call it functional medicine, others integrative medicine, still others just comprehensive medicine. It is still a new concept to many and so not well appreciated. It is contrary to how most physicians were initially trained and to what they learn in seminars and journal articles today. A single drug, device, surgery or procedure will not correct the myriad causes of today's chronic illnesses nor will it address the patient's unique personal needs. Recall again Osler's dictum, "The good physician treats the disease; the great physician treats the patient."

Most Americans do not realize how important and valuable comprehensive primary care can be to their overall health. But if you want to benefit from much better care, if you want a doctor who is not frustrated and can spend time listening to you, if you want your total costs of health care to decline rather than rise, then you need to educate yourself and then advocate. Talk to legislators, insurers, employers and especially your doctors. As Abraham Lincoln said more than a century and a half ago, "In this age, in this country, public sentiment is everything. With it, nothing can fail; against it, nothing can succeed. Whoever molds public sentiment goes deeper than he who enacts statutes, or pronounces judicial decisions."

Concerted patient action will force the issue and make change occur. It will be a win for everyone. Now is the perfect time. Congress and the president need to understand the crisis, appreciate the value of comprehensive 21st century primary care and place its resolution front and center in new legislation. It will mean better health, better medical care and lower total costs of healthcare.

Patients and PCPs will need to take charge and change the paradigm of primary care. Patients need to demand the time they deserve and a doctor who understands the concept of addressing the causes of disease, not just the symptoms of disease. PCPs need to insist that they will give the time and accept the responsibility of chronic disease specialist using a functional medicine approach.[iv]

You deserve a great doctor. Look[v] for one but recognize that you will probably have to pay at least a modest portion, likely even more, of the physician's fees out of pocket. I believe that it will be worth your money.

[iv] You can learn more from my book *Fixing the Primary Care Crisis –Reclaiming the Patient-Physician Relationship and Returning Healthcare to You and Your Doctor.*

[v] Concierge Medicine Today maintains a listing of physicians that practice using the direct primary care, membership, retainer or concierge model. https://conciergemedicinetoday.org/. The Institute for Functional Medicine maintains a listing of physicians and other providers that have participated in their training programs. https://www.ifm.org/find-a-practitioner/

CHAPTER THIRTEEN
A GREY HEAD IS A CROWN OF GLORY

"For some days now, I have had in mind a word that seems ugly: old age, a thought that frightens."
—Pope Francis on the occasion of his 80th birthday, December 17, 2016

We are all aging every day, but mostly we ignore it, do not recognize it, or even deny it. Then all of a sudden we look in the mirror and realize that older age has found us. Even then, each person deals with aging differently. Dr. Seuss parody (Chapter 1) sees nothing but adversity in aging. Others accept aging but are aware of the passing of time and the limited time left—recall the story about the 72-inch folding ruler in Chapter 1. Others, perhaps most, who recognize the changes as they come but desperately want to deny them using makeup, Botox or cosmetic surgery to fool others, if not themselves.

During adult life, most organs and body functions lose about 1 percent per year, more or less (Chapter 2). This can be slowed in a meaningful way using the seven keys detailed in the foregoing chapters—quality lifestyle modifications that include good nutrition, exercise, stress management, good sleep, no tobacco, intellectual stimulation and social engagement (Chapters 6-8).

Many, perhaps most, people are not content with lifestyle modifications and find them difficult to achieve. Instead, they want the simpler approach—a pill (Chapter 9). Only recently has some of the physiology of aging been elucidated, with much more to learn. From what is now known, new approaches may extend life, reduce age-prevalent disease and create what might be called the *longevity dividend*. The pharmaceutical industry, the biotech industry, and others are hard at work. There is a trial underway to determine the value of metformin in slowing aging and reducing chronic illnesses. Soon there may be a drug to eradicate senescent cells. Compounds similar to resveratrol, the compound in red wine that has lengthened the lives of mice, may be on the horizon. Infusing blood plasma from the young, which also was effective in mice, is being studied in humans as are other pharmaceutical approaches. One or more may have promise.

There are other individuals and companies – and not just a few – who are not content with a modest improvement in health and longevity. Instead, they're seeking a dramatic lengthening of life, perhaps immortality. They want the "Fountain of Youth" at last. Gene therapy to lengthen telomeres with enhancement of telomerase is a current example (Chapter 10).

Clearly, aging has become a serious area of study with government grant-funding, pharmaceutical activity, and venture capital encouraging entrepreneurs to address innovative concepts all coming into play. We can expect rapid advances in knowledge and multiple attempts to push back the biologic clock in coming years.

In the meantime, how will you approach aging? Is it a journey, a time of growth, or a time of diminishment? It depends on your outlook. A friend told my wife, "These small problems are annoying, aren't they? Nothing dramatic generally, but as a neurologist had put it to me almost 10 years ago about an essential tremor – which has gotten worse since then – 'It is just a benign manifestation of aging.'" Benign, perhaps, but her friend is not at all pleased to have the worsening tremor. She feels less complete, less capable than before, and diminished.

Does aging imply "diminishment?" Another friend sees it that way and offered Robert Frost's "The Oven Bird" as meaningful to her.

There is a singer everyone has heard,
Loud, a mid-summer and a mid-wood bird,
Who makes the solid tree trunks sound again.
He says that leaves are old and that for flowers
Mid-summer is to spring as one to ten.
He says the early petal-fall is past
When pear and cherry bloom went down in showers

On sunny days a moment overcast;
And comes that other fall we name the fall.
He says the highway dust is over all.
The bird would cease and be as other birds
But that he knows in singing not to sing.
The question that he frames in all but words
Is what to make of a diminished thing.

Yes, aging means less strength and mobility, reduced hearing and vision, some cognitive decline and ultimately ends with death. But there is an opportunity for much pleasure, much meaning and much value to self and others during those "elder" years. It is a good time to remember that "a grey head is a crown of glory" (Proverbs, 16:31). Aging can be a time of transformation, not just diminishment. The story of Ivan Ilyich illustrates the transformation that can occur. "The Death of Ivan Ilyich," a short novella of less than 70 pages by Leo Tolstoy, seeks to address redemption even at the very end of life.[70] Ilyich lived his life as many do—ordinary, attempting to be successful, rising to some degree of status and comfort but achieving nothing of great value. The story opens in Chapter 2 with "Ivan Ilyich's life had been most simple and most ordinary and therefore most terrible." He has scrupulously avoided thinking about why he is here, what he might wish to accomplish in his life nor has he thought about his ultimate death. Instead, he has only focused on the less important superficial issues. Now, at age 45 with an illness that assumes death is near, he realizes he has squandered his days and wishes to come to terms with the meaning of life before death. His servant – a poor man of humble status who devotes himself to helping Ivan however he can – is his new inspiration. His most valuable assistance is as an example of selflessness and spiritual richness. Ilyich slowly begins to recognize his own deficiencies and the servant's great gift and soon is transformed—just in time. These are our questions to contemplate: What choices have we made in this life? Can we – should we – adjust course?

However defined, life is a journey—including the elder years. It all depends on how you live it. Ivan Ilyich realized at the end that his choices created a journey he came to see as inadequate. My friend and colleague, Harry Oken, M.D., a superb primary care physician that I referred to earlier, writes a regular newsletter to his patients. Here is a section from one that he wrote just after he and his wife lost their beloved dog, titled *The Journey*:

> Her [their dog] leaving reminds me that everything changes and nothing remains the same. When you can learn to accept that instead of clinging to the past, it makes life a bit easier. How do you go forward in the face of loss or the adversity of challenge?
>
> Be in the moment and make the most of it. Intend to experience the next moment, next hour, next day, next week, next month and the next year, fully. It all starts with the intention to be present and mindful and then that intention turns into action and then you will get what you create. Extend kindness always. Smile whenever you can. Clear your mind with meditation, exercise daily, eat healthy, and sleep well. These healthy practices tip the scales in your favor for a longer, healthier, fuller life. We all have the same ultimate destination; when and how we get there defines the journey. If you are a sailor, you know you cannot control the direction of the wind, but you can change the position of the sails.

"Uncle John" died last year at age 101, almost 102. He had lived a long full life; his had been quite a journey. He was a member of that "greatest generation" who served in the Navy during WWII. His ship was torpedoed yet he came home to raise a family, be part of the community, build a career, and later become a grandfather and great grandfather. He brought a quiet decency yet a sense of joy to all who knew him. Despite having some clear and tragic losses, including the loss of his daughter and then his wife, he remained upbeat and resilient. He knew how and when to change the position of his sails. He sensed a purpose to life similar to the Okinawan concept of "Ikigai" and had that fundamental optimism toward life found in the Nicoya Peninsula residents' "Pura Vida" (Chapter 5). A poem, "The Dash," was read at his grave site. [71] The poem emphasizes that it is not the dates on the tomb stone that are important; rather it is the "dash." The dash represents the time of life, what the person did or did not do. The poem ends with the question, will you be pleased at how the still living will view your lifetime, your dash? With the formal service complete, while the bugler played Taps in the background, the honor guard lifted the flag from his coffin and, with loving care, folded it and passed it to the commanding officer, who in turn presented it to the grandsons with the words, "The President of the United States and the Secretary of Defense have authorized me to express their sincere appreciation for your grandfather's service to his country."

Life is what one makes of it. It is the time between birth and death; the dash. The elder years, like all of the years of life, can be rich and rewarding. It is not necessary to think as an older person that you have been cast aside. You carry great wisdom, the culture of society, the sense of who we are as a people. Even if you feel, like Ivan Ilyich, that you have not accomplished much of value or meaning, there is still time. It is never too late to begin with a transformed life.

...

Perhaps science will advance so telomere reconstitution is a practical reality, DNA epigenetic changes can be reversed, senescent cells can be eradicated, free radical damage to mitochondria can be dismantled, and the microbiome can be altered back to a youthful status. Perhaps metformin or resveratrol or some other drugs will have a significant impact. Perhaps gene therapy will prove an outstanding success.

Perhaps.

But for now, it might be a more fruitful and meaningful personal use of your time and energy to consider what the normal aging process means, not only physically and mentally but also spiritually. Consider adjustments to lifestyle, behaviors and thought processes that will help usher in a productive, meaningful and healthy later years. You can do it. It will take time and effort, but the outcome will be worth it. Unlike that utterance of the Pope on his 80th birthday, *old age need not be an ugly word nor a thought that frightens.*

APPENDIX

Here is a summary review of the seven keys to increase longevity, decrease the likelihood of chronic diseases, and remain healthy. See the appropriate chapters for more detail.

An important note and disclaimer: The entire book is meant for education and in no way should be thought of as personal medical advice. It is truly critical for you to discuss any plans with your personal physician. It is quite possible that some of the suggestions made here would not be appropriate for you.

Nutrition

Seniors (along with anyone who is overweight) need a nutrient-dense but calorie-lite diet plan. A good basis is the Mediterranean diet.

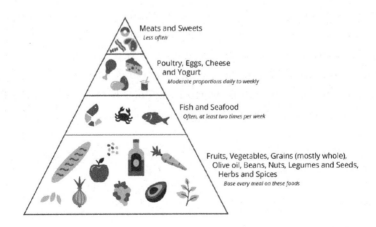

Recall that at the base of the pyramid are large quantities of multiple types and colors of vegetables, lots of green leafies (kale, spinach, arugula, Swiss chard, dandelion) and fruits. These are heavy in nutrients, low in calories and contain plenty of fiber for the gut microbiota. Fresh or frozen berries (such as strawberries, blueberries, blackberries) also have high levels of valuable polyphenols.

- Two-thirds of your plate should be covered with vegetables. Include a good salad of dark green leafies to top it off nicely. Use olive oil with a vinegar or lemon as salad dressing.

- The diet calls for *whole* grains, which means no refined white flour and thus no breads, cereals, pastas, cakes, pies, cookies or pizza made from white flour. If you want to go further still, eliminate gluten from your diet.

- Beans and lentils are also on the base of the diet and can be a good meat replacement a few times per week since they contain multiple proteins, fiber and vitamins and minerals.

- Nuts and seeds contain healthy fats and can be eaten in abundance as can avocados. Olive oil is the oil of choice.

- The next layer up is fish, especially fin fish with high concentrations of omega-3 fatty acids and valuable proteins.

- Dairy and poultry are next up the pyramid. Look for eggs from free range chickens and likewise look for slaughtered chickens that were range fed.

- Above poultry on the pyramid are meats in limited quantities. Serving sizes should be about the size of a deck of cards. Buy meats from grass-fed steers and sheep, not animals penned and fed grains to make them fat.

- At the very top of the pyramid is sugar. Avoid it. That means not just avoiding it in your coffee and tea but reading labels in the store where all number of goods have added sugars. Remember that women should have no more than 25 grams of sugar per day and men no more than 37 grams. One 12-ounce can of most sodas exceeds a woman's limit.

- Buy organic where possible. It costs more but may be worth the expense.

Exercise & Movement

Aerobic Exercise

- Walk, swim, or cycle five or six days each week for 30 to 40 minutes.
- Walking at a steady pace on a level path is sufficient.
- If you stop to chat or take in a sight, add on makeup time.
- You can boost your metabolism by following the High Intensity Interval Training (HIIT) program. Reread the details in Chapter 7.
- Engage in resistance exercise (weights).
- Work all muscle groups 2-3 times per week.
- Repeat each weight 8-12 times, rest and repeat again two more times
- You can do some basic resistance exercises at home with sit-ups, pushups, squats, and "the plank." These are great for developing the core muscles. But to work all muscle groups, it is advisable to go to a fitness center and use the various nautilus-type machines. These are generally safe and effective.

Balance Exercises

Balance depends on eyesight, the semicircular canals in our inner ears, and our ability to sense where our joints are positioned through proprioception nerves. All three decline with age, so all three need practice together.

- Test yourself with heel-to-toe walking for 20 feet. Then do some simple balance exercises at least twice a week.
- For example, stand a foot or so from a wall, with feet 12 inches apart. Touch the wall with your fingertips. When you feel well balanced, with weight balanced over the balls and heels of each foot, drop your hands to your sides. You are using all three balance mechanisms. Hold this for 30 seconds and then continue with your eyes closed, which reduces you to just two mechanisms.
- Next, do the same exercise with your feet about three inches apart.
- Next, do the same exercise with one foot forward and one back, then reverse foot positions.
- You will find that your balance improves quickly with these exercises, dramatically reducing the chances of a fall.

Chronic Stress Relief

Look for ways to reduce your stressors.
- Commit to no more than you can comfortably accomplish.
- Keep some free time truly free, and don't overschedule.

Ways to Relieve Stress
- Slow deep breathing—something you can do anytime and anyplace.
- Meditation—consider downloading a few meditation aids
- Yoga—simple stretching (Hatha yoga) or more complex work with an instructor
- Benson relaxation method—in essence, this is a simplified form of meditation that anyone can do without formal instruction or effort.
- Exercise—helps to burn off those "negative" chemicals.
- Forgive those who have harmed you in whatever manner. Don't carry it around because it will weigh you down. Life is too precious to have it consumed by your angers.

Sleep Hygiene

- Try to obtain about eight hours of sleep each night.
- Use your bedroom only for sleep, not for watching television, or looking at your smart phone to check emails or look at Facebook.
- Your bedroom should be dark. Get blackout shades for windows, turn off all lights including smart phones and your clock face.
- Keep to a regular schedule of retiring and arising.
- Some relaxing music before bedtime may be helpful.
- Just before dozing off, think about gratitude and thankfulness.
- Consider melatonin an hour before bed, if necessary.
- Avoid violent, horror and other excitatory television shows before bedtime. If you must watch TV, watch humor instead.
- Similarly, don't read books or articles before bedtime that are "downers."

Tobacco

- None.

Intellectual Challenges

- Learn a new dance step, a new language, a new musical instrument.
- Do something creative, such as art or music.
- Engage in a hobby that requires concentration, such as chess.
- Take a challenging course and test yourself.
- Consider "brain games" from the internet.

Social Engagement

- Make and keep friends.
- Get involved with your church, synagogue, mosque or other religious group.
- Join a book club or other group that interacts regularly.
- Frequent the local senior center and get involved.

Purpose in Life

This is above and beyond the seven keys but can be very valuable.

Recall from the discussion of the Blue Zones that the Okinawans had a concept they call "Ikigai," which literally is a combination of the words "life" and "value." And in the Nicoya Peninsula of Costa Rico, they refer to a spirit of "Pura Vida" or "Pure Life," which is a fundamental optimism toward life.

Stop and think (meditate) about your life's purpose. This is not necessarily the same as your career since that likely ends at retirement. Your purpose may change over time and it need not be to change the world, become a business success or become famous, but something much more basic. Understanding it will offer you peace of mind and a reason to get up each morning.

...

A few additional considerations...

Oral Hygiene

- Be sure to have a dental exam twice per year and a prophylaxis twice per year.

Driving

- Don't drive distracted – texting, cell phone or even fiddling with the radio. Watch the road.
- Don't drink and drive.

About Supplements and Vitamins

- First and foremost, they are just that – supplements – and not to be confused with a replacement for the *7 Keys*. Proper lifestyle modifications are the essential ingredients, with that proviso that you need to discuss any vitamin, mineral and supplement program with your physician.
- Most people will benefit from a high quality, full potency multivitamin daily.
- Those living in a temperate climate often get too little sunshine and so require vitamin D supplements. Get your blood tested and adjust based on the doctor's advice.
- Many older individuals absorb vitamin B12 less well than younger individuals. Get tested and supplement as indicated.
- Other supplements that may be useful on a case by case basis are:
  A high potency B complex combination.
  Antioxidant vitamins such A, C, E, Coenzyme Q10
  The minerals Magnesium, Zinc, Selenium
- Many herbs and spices have healthy attributes in addition to making meals more enjoyable.

About Screening Tests

- The most important screening tests are height and weight or waist size and height. The first can be used to calculate body mass index (BMI) and the second to assure that your waist circumference is less than your height in inches.
- Blood pressure and pulse are important as is cholesterol and glucose (blood sugar) screening.
- Other screening should be done based only after a discussion with your physician and considering the pro and cons of each—value, cost, downsides given your personal situation, including age.

About Vaccines for those Over 65

- These can be lifesaving or prevent substantial debility.
- Influenza yearly.
- Pneumococcal ("Pneumonia") vaccine every five years. There are two types; get both.
- Tetanus and diphtheria every ten years.
- Shingles (zoster) vaccine. Obtain the new version from Glaxo even if you received the Merck vaccine in the past. The new vaccine is more effective and lasts longer.

ABOUT THE AUTHOR

Stephen C. Schimpff, MD MACP is a graduate of Rutgers University and Yale University School of Medicine with a career that spans over fifty years. He is a quasi-retired internist, researcher, clinical professor of medicine at the University of Maryland School of Medicine and former professor of public policy in the School of Public Policy, founding director of the University of Maryland Greenebaum Cancer Center, and former University of Maryland Medical Center chief executive officer. He is board certified in internal medicine, medical oncology and infectious diseases. He was recently elevated to Master, the highest honor bestowed by the American College of Physicians. His early career was first at the National Cancer Institute and then the University of Maryland Medical School where his research on preventing and treating infections in seriously ill cancer patients became acclaimed worldwide. He joined the University of Maryland Medical System as chief operating officer and later as chief executive officer of the flagship University of Maryland Medical Center. He has authored or co-authored five books for the general public on medical topics, and co-authored a history of Canaan Valley, WV. He and Carol, his wife of over 54 years, live in Maryland.

Learn more about Dr. Schimpff's books, articles and blog at: www.medicalmegatrends.com

ACKNOWLEDGEMENTS

The seeds of this book began with an invitation from Geary Milliken, President & CEO of Lutheran Village at Millers Grant and his associates to speak at two venues on "Aging Gracefully." Expecting a dozen or so, I was surprised at a turnout of well over 100 who greeted the talks with enthusiasm and many questions. This led to a newspaper interview and then an invitation from Ron Carlson, former senior executive with the U.S. Public Health Service and current chair of the Paul R. Willging Endowment to present the Endowment's lecture on aging to another larger audience. The interest demonstrated a widespread desire for information and hence this book.

Many people offered suggestions and specific guidance over the past three years. Among them are academic gerontologists Jack M. Guralnik, MD, PhD, Steven Gambert, MD and Jacob Blumenthal MD, along with Genomics Institute director Claire Fraser, PhD each at the University of Maryland Medical School, whose lectures began my quest to learn more. Andy Lazris, MD a practicing gerontologist and author of *Curing Medicare* and Matt Narrett, MD, gerontologist and chief medical officer at continuing care retirement community operator Erickson Living were frequent advisors and ongoing supporters. Harry Oken, MD, a practicing primary care physician, advised me on diet and exercise based on his courses for the Columbia Association. My personal primary care physician, Gary Milles, MD, was most helpful as was Lou Grimmel, Sr., CEO of long term care Lorien Health Services. John Erickson, founder of Erickson Living and developer of its 19 continuing care retirement communities, was an early mentor. David Miller, PhD, friend and coauthor of an earlier book, told me the story of the 72- inch ruler found in Chapter 1. Physical Therapist Frank Jannotta first taught me about muscle wasting with aging.

The Charlestown Retirement Community resident life director, Sherry Parrish, MSW, and TV studio director Thomas Moore enlisted me to do a weekly health and wellness show for the in-house TV channel available to the 2000 residents. Carol Jones, RN a retired public health nurse and I created 14 half hour episodes on the topics in this book and shortened versions were placed on YouTube complements of Moore and the station staff—Michael Woodard and Konstantinos Viennas. Resident comments from those shows helped to make the text more complete.

Our daughter Becky Schimpff, having visited one of the Blue Zones twice, was very helpful with that chapter.

Multiple colleagues, friends and family – too many to name – were ready and willing to assist as requested.

Margaret Frazier converted my dictations to type and later formatted the text and end notes. The Charlestown Writers Critique Group read each chapter as they progressed and offered insightful suggestions. Journalist Carolyn Crist copyedited the manuscript. Ken Lundeen, friend and outstanding lawyer, proofread the entire manuscript; amazing what others (including me) missed and he found.

Sage Growth Partners including its CEO, Dan D'Orizo have been constant supporters. Sage campaign manager Alex Lucas, with assistance from Sarah Koch, created the internal graphics for which I am most grateful. They greatly improve the readability of the text.

Larry Gerrans, CEO of Sanovas, Inc., was an early encourager of this project and offered frequent advice.

Lou Moriconi, as he has done for my previous books, envisioned and then developed the cover design. First impressions are critical, and he has certainly led the way.

My literary agent, Cynthia Zigmund, Second City Publishing Services LLC, offered advice and encouragement over the time this book was under preparation and guided the placement for publication.

Despite all of this advice, encouragement and specific actions by others, any errors are mine alone.

Most importantly, I thank Carol Schimpff, my wife of over 54 years, for her interest, encouragement and even prodding to bring this project to fruition. She has constantly, for all these years, provided the inspiration for me to do my best yet find balance with reflection and enjoyment of family and nature.

EXCERPT FROM THE 21ST CENTURY PLAGUE: THE SCOURGE OF COMPLEX CHRONIC DISEASES

COMING SOON FROM STEPHEN C SCHIMPFF, MD, MACP

The Plague or Black Death reduced the population of Europe by about a third between 1347 and 1350. The cause, a bacterial infection in fleas carried on the backs of rats, was unknown. Today there is a new plague that is systematically robbing us of health and longevity. These chronic diseases cause most deaths today and consume most of the healthcare dollar. The serious diseases of today are markedly different than in years past. Decades ago, most illnesses were acute (or temporary, such as pneumonia and appendicitis), but today the vast majority are chronic and persist, as of now, for life. What is this transition and how did it occur?

The 21st Century Plague is the spectrum of complex chronic diseases such as diabetes, heart failure, emphysema, cancer, multiple sclerosis, celiac disease, Crohn's disease, lupus erythematosus and rheumatoid arthritis and, the most dreaded of all, Alzheimer's disease. Chronic disease is transforming health, medical costs, and the delivery of care. Once developed, they usually last a lifetime, are difficult to manage and usually are expensive to treat. Chronic illnesses, once rare, are becoming commonplace. They are responsible for the vast majority of disability and most mortality, as well as most of today's very high health care costs. But, notably, most are preventable.

Chronic illnesses have three primary antecedents: genetics, aging and lifestyle.

Most chronic diseases occur in individuals predisposed through their genes, but genes do not imply destiny. The gene only becomes active (or expressed) if triggered. Usually the trigger comes from the environment such as what you eat, drink or breathe.

Chronic disease prevalence rises sharply with older age. Researchers debate whether aging causes this increase or whether a long life allows the disease to manifest.

Adverse behaviors are by far the major causes of most chronic illnesses. The key negative lifestyle factors include tobacco, adverse diet, low activity, high stress, limited sleep, excessive alcohol, along with inadequate dental hygiene, and careless actions – such as texting while driving.

. . .

Our medical care system has developed over centuries around the process of diagnosing and treating acute illnesses such as pneumonia, a gall bladder attack or appendicitis. The internist gives an antibiotic for the pneumonia and the patient gets better. The surgeon cuts out the gall bladder or the appendix and the patient is cured. One patient, one doctor. However, patients with chronic illnesses need a different approach to care. They need long-term care, not episodic care. They need a doctor who attends to the care of their chronic illnesses with intensity. Often, they need the primary care physician (PCP) to enlist a multi-disciplinary, team-based approach with the PCP serving as the orchestrator managing the myriad physician specialists, nurse practitioners, health coaches, nutritionists, pharmacists, and nurses. This manager should also review all tests and procedures to create a unified, coordinated care approach.

Importantly, this physician should be trained and up-to-date in the management of these chronic illnesses, not just the symptoms, but the underlying causes—of which much more will be written in the following chapters. Attending "to the patient with a disease" along with the root causes of the disease rather than just the disease and its symptoms will be critical. To do this, the U.S. health care system will need a new style of care and great intensity to help these patients, improve their care, and reduce total costs. It can be done and is being done by some physicians and teams today. Even more, it can be expanded to the entire population. It will cost more money up front, but the total costs of care will be immediately and significantly reduced, and with the addition of good preventive techniques, the long-term costs will decrease dramatically. The important result, of course, is not money but health and wellness, returning individuals to good health and maintaining others in a wellness state for years to come.

The number of patients under care by each PCP needs to be reduced to no more than 500-800 rather than the current 2,500-3,000 patients. At this lower level, the provider can have the time needed to listen, prevent, diagnose, treat and think. This will allow doctors to effectively manage the care of patients with chronic illnesses. It will also reduce the excessive use of specialists, tests and procedures, and the reflex to hand out a prescription when a lifestyle change would be both more appropriate and more effective. The end result will be better health and lower total costs.

The future must include a larger focus on wellness, health promotion and preventive medicine. A shift to a new model of care – one effective for chronic illness rather than acute or episodic illness – will substantially improve quality, bolster patient and physician satisfaction, and dramatically reduce costs. It actually is possible to improve quality care yet reduce the costs of care, while improving patient satisfaction and reducing provider frustration. This requires a new paradigm in management, incentives and compensation for physicians, and new responsibilities and incentives for patients as well.

END NOTES

[1] Luhby, T., America's richest men live 15 years longer than poor men, CNN Money, April 11, 2016 http://money.cnn.com/2016/04/11/news/economy/life-expectancy-rich-poor/index.html Last accessed Oct 25, 2017

[2] Jones, D, Podolsky, M and Greene, J, The burden of disease and the changing task of medicine, New Engl. J Med 2012; 366:2333-2338

[3] McGinnis, J and Foege, W, Actual causes of death in the United States. JAMA. 1993: 270:2207-2212

[4] Jones, DS and Greene, J, Is Dementia in Decline? Historical Trends and Future Trajectories, New Engl J Med, 2106; 374: 507-509 http://www.nejm.org/doi/full/10.1056/NEJMp1514434 Last accessed Oct 25, 2017

[5] Fossel, M., Cells, Aging, and Human Disease, Oxford Univ Press, 2004

[6] Vincent, GK and Velkof, VA, The next four decades-The older population in the United States, 2010-2050, May, 2010 US Census Department https://www.census.gov/prod/2010pubs/p25-1138.pdf *Last accessed Oct 25, 2017*

[7] Bergen, G, Stevens, M, Burns, E, Falls and Fall Injuries Among Adults Aged ≥65 Years—United States, 2014, Morbidity and Mortality Weekly Reports, September 23, 2016 / 65(37);993–998 http://www.cdc.gov/mmwr/volumes/65/wr/mm6537a2.htm?s_cid=mm6537a2_w *Last accessed Oct 25, 2017*

[8] Belsky, BW, etal, Quantification of biological aging in young adults, Proceeding of the National Academy of Sciences, July 6, 2015, E4104-4110 http://www.pnas.org/content/112/30/E4104.full Last *accessed Oct 25, 2017*

[9] Lopex-Otin, C, Galuzzi, L, Freije, J, and Kroemer, G, Metabolic Control of Longevity, Cell, 166: 802-821, 2016, http://dx.doi.org/10.1016/j.cell.2016.07.031 Last accessed October 25 2017

[10] Labbadia, J, Morimoto, R., Repression of the Heat Shock Response Is a Programmed Event at the Onset of Reproduction. *Molecular Cell*, 2015; DOI: 10.1016/j.molcel.2015.06.027 Last accessed Oct 25, 2017

[11] Northwestern University, "Simple flip of genetic switch determines aging or longevity in animals: Scientists pinpoint start of aging, discover it is not a slow series of random events." ScienceDaily, 23 July 2015. www.sciencedaily.com/releases/2015/07/150723125244.htm Last accessed Oct 25, 2017

[12] Hashizume, O, et al, Epigenetic regulation of the nuclear-coded GCAT and SHMT2 genes confers human age-associated mitochondrial respiration defects. *Scientific Reports*, 2015; 5: https://www.nature.com/articles/srep10434 Last accessed Oct 25, 2017

[13] A reasonably comprehensive article by Ben Best in Life Extension Magazine in November, 2015 reviews the microbiome and aging issues. http://www.lifeextension.com/magazine/2015/11/the-microbiome-of-aging-and-age-related-disease-conference/page-01 Last accessed August 30, 2016

[14] Zapata HJ[1], Quagliarello VJ, The microbiota and microbiome in aging: potential implications in health and age-related diseases, J Am Geriatr Soc, 2015; Apr;63(4):776-81, https://www.ncbi.nlm.nih.gov/pubmed/25851728 Last accessed November 4, 2017

[15] Yong, E, Clearing the Body's Retired Cells Slows Aging and Extends Life, The Atlantic, Feb 6, 2016   http://www.theatlantic.com/science/archive/2016/02/clearing-retired-cells-extends-life/459723/   Last accessed November 4, 2017

[16] Baker, DJ, etal, Clearance of p16[Ink4a]-positive senescent cells delays ageing-associated disorders, Nature, 2011, 479: 232–236. http://www.ncbi.nlm.nih.gov/pmc/articles/PMC3468323/ November 4, 2017

[17] Unity Biotechnology web site http://unitybiotechnology.com/ November 4, 2017

[18] Sent by a friend; original source unknown

[19] Schmidt, E, Epigenetic clock predicts life expectancy, UCLA Newsroom, September 28, 2016, http://newsroom.ucla.edu/releases/epigenetic-clock-predicts-life-expectancy-ucla-led-study-shows Last accessed October 25, 2017

[20] Marioni, RE, etal DNA methylation age of blood predicts all-cause mortality in later life, Genome Biol. 2015; 16(1): 25. http://genomebiology.biomedcentral.com/articles/10.1186/s13059-015-0584-6 Last accessed October 25, 2017

[21] Gibbs, W.W, And Aging: The Clock Watcher, Nature, April 8, 2014 http://www.nature.com/news/biomarkers-and-ageing-the-clock-watcher-1.15014 Last accessed October 25, 2017

[22] Schmidt, E., Epigenetic clock predicts life expectancy, UCLA-led study shows, UCLA Newsroom, Sept 28, 2016, http://newsroom.ucla.edu/releases/epigenetic-clock-predicts-life-expectancy-ucla-led-study-shows Last accessed October 25, 2017

[23] Buettner, D, The Blue Zones, Second Edition: 9 Lessons for Living Longer From the People Who've Lived the Longest, National Geographic, 2012

[24] *Poulain, M; Pes, G; Grasland, C; Carru, C; Ferrucci, L; Baggio, G; Franceschi, C; Deiana, L,* Identification of a geographic area characterized by extreme longevity in the Sardinia island: the AKEA study. *Experimental Gerontology, 2004; 39 (9): 1423–1429.* http://www.sciencedirect.com/science/article/pii/S0531556504002141 . *Last accessed November 2, 2017*

[25] Buettner, D, "Longevity, The Secrets of Long Life - National Geographic Magazine". *2005 Last accessed November 2, 2017*

[26] Buettner, D, The Blue Zones – Lessons for living longer from the people who've lived the longest, National Geographic, 2008

[27] Rousseau, B, Rosemary and time: does this Italian hamlet have a recipe for long life?, New York Times, Oct. 19, 2016, https://www.nytimes.com/2016/10/20/world/what-in-the-world/rosemary-and-time-does-this-italian-hamlet-have-a-recipe-for-long-life.html *Last accessed November 2, 2017*

[28] Loma Linda University, Adventist Health Study -2, https://publichealth.llu.edu/adventist-health-studies/about Last accessed November 13, 2017

[29] Orlich, M, etal, Vegetarian dietary patterns and mortality in Adventist health study 2, JAMA Intern Med, 2013: 173: 1230-38 https://

jamanetwork.com/journals/jamainternalmedicine/fullarticle/1710093 Last accessed November 2, 2017

30 Khera, A.V., etal, Genetic Risk, Adherence to a Healthy Lifestyle, and Coronary Disease, N Engl J Med 2016; 375:2349-2358 http://www.nejm.org/doi/full/10.1056/NEJMoa1605086?query=featured_home Last Accessed Oct 25 2017

31 Oaklander, M., The New Science of Exercise, Time Health, Sept 12, 2016, http://time.com/4475628/the-new-science-of-exercise/ Last accessed November 2, 2017

32 Austad, S, A Young Field about Growing Older: Six Ways Research Is Changing How We Age, Huffington Post, October 12, 2016, http://www.huffingtonpost.com/american-federation-for-aging-research/a-young-field-about-growi_b_12455050.html? Last accessed November 2, 2017

33 Eijsvogels, TMH, Exercise is medicine: at any dose? J of the Amer Med Assoc, 2015; 314: 1915-1916

34 Jha P., etal, 21st-Century Hazards of Smoking and Benefits of Cessation in the United States, N Engl J Med 2013; 368:341-350, 2013 http://www.nejm.org/doi/full/10.1056/NEJMsa1211128 Last accessed November 2, 2017

35 How Aging Affects Driving, NIH Senior Health, available at this site https://nihseniorhealth.gov/olderdrivers/howagingaffectsdriving/01.html Last accessed November 2, 2017

36 English poet Rose Milligan; first published on September 15th 1998 in the 21st edition of *The Lady,* England's longest running magazine for women. Readily available on the Internet

37 Russell, D, Peplau, L, Cutrona, C, The revised UCLA loneliness scale: concurrent and discriminant validity evidence, J of Personality and Social Psychology, 1980; 39: 472-480

38 Small, G, 2 weeks to a younger brain – an innovative program for a better memory and sharper mind, Humanix Books, 2016

39 Gibala, M quoted by M Outlander in The New Science of Exercise, Time, Sept 12, 2016, http://time.com/4475628/the-new-science-of-exercise/ Last accessed October 12, 2017

40 Forbes D, Forbes SC, Blake CM, Thiessen EJ, Forbes S, Exercise programs for people with dementia, April 15, 2015, http://www.cochrane.org/

CD006489/DEMENTIA_exercise-programs-for-people-with-dementia Last accessed October 12, 2017

[41] Isaacson, R, and Ochner, C, The Alzheimer's prevention and treatment diet – using nutrition to combat the effects of Alzheimer's disease, SquareOne, 2016

[42] Bredesen, D, The end of Alzheimer's – the first program to prevent and reverse cognitive decline, Avery Books, 2017

[43] Bredesen, D, Reversal of cognitive decline: a novel therapeutic program, Aging 2014; 6: 707-717 https://doi.org/10.18632/aging.100690 Last accessed October 12, 2017

[44] Olshansky, J, Martin, G and Kirkland, J., "Aging: The Longevity Dividend" Cold Spring Harbor Laboratory Press, 2015

[45] Brody, Jane, Finding a Drug for Healthy Aging, New York Times, February 1, 2016. http://well.blogs.nytimes.com/2016/02/01/pursuing-the-dream-of-healthy-aging/?_r=1 Last accessed November 3, 2017

[46] Brody, Jane, Finding a Drug for Healthy Aging, New York Times, February 1, 2016. http://well.blogs.nytimes.com/2016/02/01/pursuing-the-dream-of-healthy-aging/?_r=1 Last accessed November 3, 2017

[47] Thomas, N, et al, Glutathione maintenance mitigates age-related susceptibility to redox cycling agents, *Redox Biology* (2016). DOI: 10.1016/j.redox.2016.09.010

[48] Hubbard, BP, etal,   Evidence for a Common Mechanism of SIRT1 Regulation by Allosteric Activators, Science, Vol 339, Issue 6124, 08 March 2013 http://science.sciencemag.org/content/339/6124/1216?sid=b369173a-02a4-4f5c-b693-4a1e4e870a4d Last accessed November 3, 2017

[49] Forslund, K, etal, Nature, 2015; 528: 262

[50] Leslie, M, Whatever happened to..., Science, 16 September 2016; 353:1198-1201

[51] Pearl, M, The Blood of Young People Won't Help Peter Thiel Fight Death, Science Alert, August 5, 2016 http://www.sciencealert.com/here-s-everything-scientists-know-about-how-to-avoid-ageing Last accessed November 3, 2017

[52] Jocelyn Kaiser, Antiaging trial using young blood stirs concerns, Science, August 5 2016, 353; 537-8

[53] Male hormone reverses cell aging in clinical trial, Eureka Alert, July 25, 2016, http://www.eurekalert.org/pub_releases/2016-07/fda-mhr072516.php Last accessed November 3, 2017

Danielle M. Townsley, M.D, etal, Danazol Treatment for Telomere Diseases, N Engl J Med 2016; 374:1922-1931,http://www.nejm.org/doi/full/10.1056/NEJMoa1515319 Last accessed November 3, 2017

and an accompanying editorial

Lansdorp, P.M., Telomeres on Steroids—Turning Back the Mitotic Clock?, N Engl J Med 2016; 374:1978-1980 http://www.nejm.org/doi/full/10.1056/NEJMe1602822 Last accessed November 3, 2017

[54] Handelsman, DJ, Testosterone and male aging: faltering hope for rejuvenation, J Amer Med Assoc, 2017; 317: 699-700

[55] Mittendorf, J, and Sagan, D, Cracking The Aging Code: The New Science Of Growing Old – And What It Means For Staying Young, Flatiron Books, June 14, 2016

[56] Cha, A., Peter Thiel's quest to find the key to eternal life, The Washington Post, April 3, 2015. https://www.washingtonpost.com/business/on-leadership/peter-thiels-life-goal-to-extend-our-time-on-this-earth/2015/04/03/b7a1779c-4814-11e4-891d-713f052086a0_story.html Last accessed November 3, 2017

[57] BioViva web site https://bioviva-science.com/ Last accessed November 3, 2017

[58] Butler, R. N. (1969). "Age-ism: Another form of bigotry". The Gerontologist. 9 (4): 243–246. doi:10.1093/geront/9.4_part_1.243

[59] Spar, D, Aging and my beauty dilemma, New York Times, Sept 24, 2016, http://www.nytimes.com/2016/09/25/fashion/aging-plastic-surgery-feminism.html

[60] Leland, J., The Wisdom of the Aged, New York Times Dec 25, 2015 http://www.nytimes.com/2015/12/27/nyregion/the-wisdom-of-the-aged.html?smid=li-share&_r=1

[61] Landry, R, Who Will Write Your Aging Story http://clvillage.org/landry-top-ten/

[62] Bahrampour, T, We are lucky if we get to be old" Washington Post, Jan 23, 2016 https://www.washingtonpost.com/local/social-issues/were-lucky-if-we-get-to-be-old-physician-and-professor-believes/2016/01/2

3/251ed8b2-b9c2-11e5-829c-26ffb874a18d_story.html?utm_term=.
e5965e910e8e

63 Gurian, M, The wonder of aging – a new approach to embracing life after
fifty, Atria Books, 2013

64 Gurian, The wonder of aging – a new approach to embracing life after
fifty

65 The life review letter was developed by faculty at Stanford University
Medical Center https://med.stanford.edu/letter/friendsandfamily.html

66 The life review letter - template is available on line at http://dearfamily.
dear-doc.appspot.com/html/healthyletter.html

67 Erickson, M, Narrett, M, Kung, J, and Davila, L, Old is the new young,
GPP Life, 2009

68 Erickson, Old is the new young

69 Schimpff, S., fixing the primary care crisis – reclaiming the patient-
physician relationship and returning healthcare decisions to you and your
doctor, CreateSpace, 2016

70 Tolstoy, Leo, The death of Ivan Ilyich, original in Russian published in
1886, English translation by Pevear, R, and Volokhonsky, L, Vintage
Classics, 2012

71 Ellis, L., "The Dash," 1996. Copyright restrictions prevent reproducing
the entire poem but it can be readily found on the Internet.

INDEX

95165890R00114

Made in the USA
Columbia, SC
12 May 2018